ATS-133   ADMISSION TEST SERIES

*This is your
PASSBOOK for...*

Funeral Service National Board Examination (FSNBE)

*Test Preparation Study Guide
Questions & Answers*

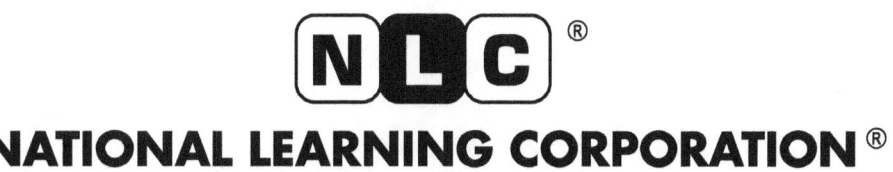

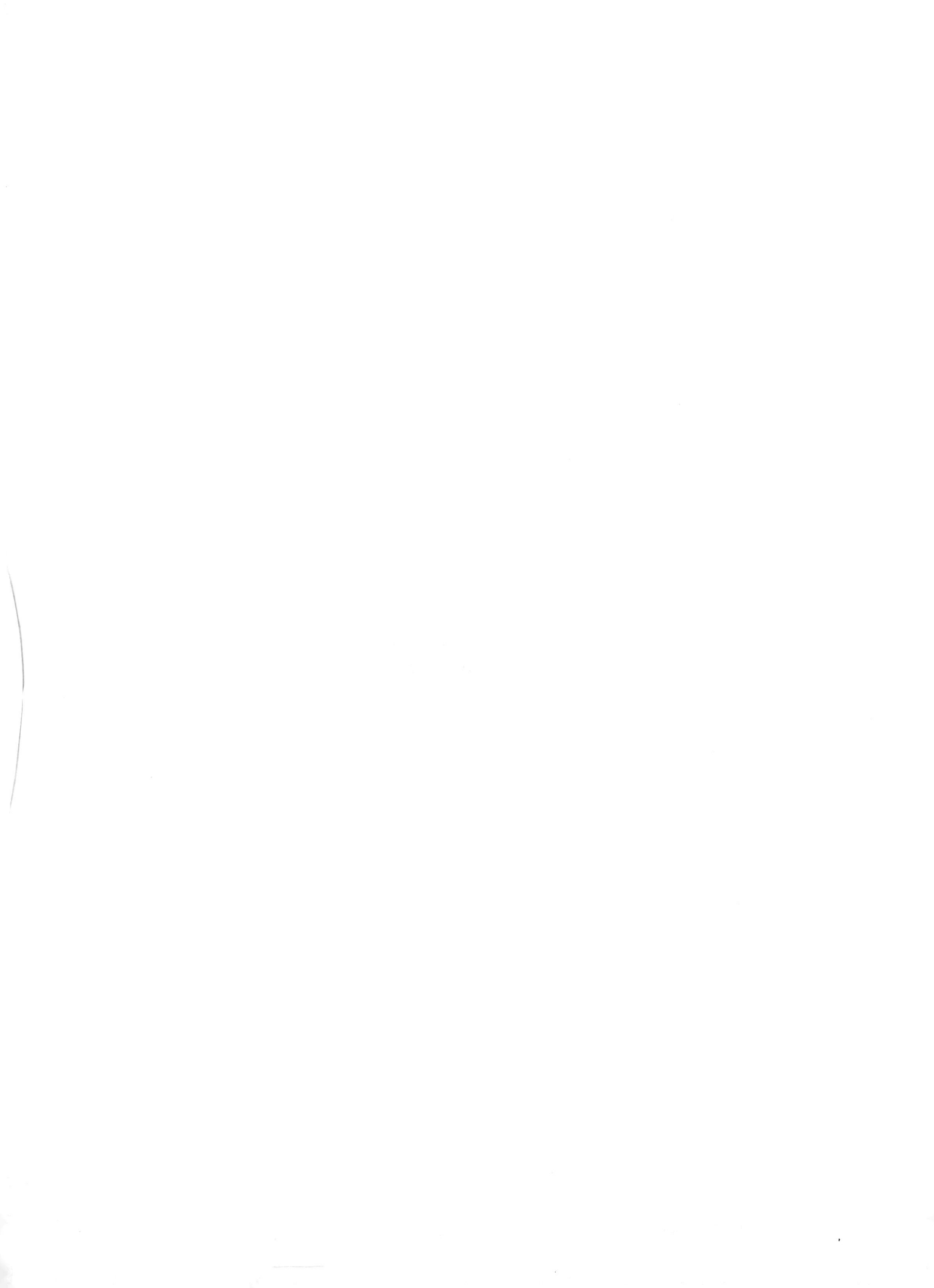

COPYRIGHT NOTICE

This book is SOLELY intended for, is sold ONLY to, and its use is RESTRICTED to individual, bona fide applicants or candidates who qualify by virtue of having seriously filed applications for appropriate license, certificate, professional and/or promotional advancement, higher school matriculation, scholarship, or other legitimate requirements of education and/or governmental authorities.

This book is NOT intended for use, class instruction, tutoring, training, duplication, copying, reprinting, excerption, or adaptation, etc., by:

1) Other publishers
2) Proprietors and/or Instructors of "Coaching" and/or Preparatory Courses
3) Personnel and/or Training Divisions of commercial, industrial, and governmental organizations
4) Schools, colleges, or universities and/or their departments and staffs, including teachers and other personnel
5) Testing Agencies or Bureaus
6) Study groups which seek by the purchase of a single volume to copy and/or duplicate and/or adapt this material for use by the group as a whole without having purchased individual volumes for each of the members of the group
7) Et al.

Such persons would be in violation of appropriate Federal and State statutes.

PROVISION OF LICENSING AGREEMENTS – Recognized educational, commercial, industrial, and governmental institutions and organizations, and others legitimately engaged in educational pursuits, including training, testing, and measurement activities, may address request for a licensing agreement to the copyright owners, who will determine whether, and under what conditions, including fees and charges, the materials in this book may be used them. In other words, a licensing facility exists for the legitimate use of the material in this book on other than an individual basis. However, it is asseverated and affirmed here that the material in this book CANNOT be used without the receipt of the express permission of such a licensing agreement from the Publishers. Inquiries re licensing should be addressed to the company, attention rights and permissions department.

All rights reserved, including the right of reproduction in whole or in part, in any form or by any means, electronic or mechanical, including photocopying, recording, or by any information storage and retrieval system, without permission in writing from the Publisher.

Copyright © 2025 by
National Learning Corporation

212 Michael Drive, Syosset, NY 11791
(516) 921-8888 • www.passbooks.com
E-mail: info@passbooks.com

PASSBOOK® SERIES

THE *PASSBOOK® SERIES* has been created to prepare applicants and candidates for the ultimate academic battlefield – the examination room.

At some time in our lives, each and every one of us may be required to take an examination – for validation, matriculation, admission, qualification, registration, certification, or licensure.

Based on the assumption that every applicant or candidate has met the basic formal educational standards, has taken the required number of courses, and read the necessary texts, the *PASSBOOK® SERIES* furnishes the one special preparation which may assure passing with confidence, instead of failing with insecurity. Examination questions – together with answers – are furnished as the basic vehicle for study so that the mysteries of the examination and its compounding difficulties may be eliminated or diminished by a sure method.

This book is meant to help you pass your examination provided that you qualify and are serious in your objective.

The entire field is reviewed through the huge store of content information which is succinctly presented through a provocative and challenging approach – the question-and-answer method.

A climate of success is established by furnishing the correct answers at the end of each test.

You soon learn to recognize types of questions, forms of questions, and patterns of questioning. You may even begin to anticipate expected outcomes.

You perceive that many questions are repeated or adapted so that you can gain acute insights, which may enable you to score many sure points.

You learn how to confront new questions, or types of questions, and to attack them confidently and work out the correct answers.

You note objectives and emphases, and recognize pitfalls and dangers, so that you may make positive educational adjustments.

Moreover, you are kept fully informed in relation to new concepts, methods, practices, and directions in the field.

You discover that you are actually taking the examination all the time: you are preparing for the examination by "taking" an examination, not by reading extraneous and/or supererogatory textbooks.

In short, this PASSBOOK®, used directedly, should be an important factor in helping you to pass your test.

FUNERAL SERVICE NATIONAL BOARD EXAMINATION (FSNBE)

The Funeral Service National Board Examination (FSNBE) provides state licensing boards and bureaus with a national evaluation of an applicant for licensure in the field of funeral service. The Exam is used in all states except California, and serves as an assessment of knowledge in the arts and sciences of a licensed funeral director or embalmer.

The FSNBE contains two separate sections – Arts and Sciences – each numbering 170 items. The Arts section is broken down into a set number of subtests and a corresponding number of questions:

Sociology/Funeral Service History	21 items
Psychology	21
Funeral Directing	27
Business Law	24
Funeral Service Law	21
Funeral Service Merchandising	21
Accounting/Computers	15
Pretest Items	20

The Sciences section is broken down as follows:

Embalming	36 items
Restorative Art	36
Microbiology	18
Pathology	24
Chemistry	18
Anatomy	18
Pretest Items	20

The exam is scored based on the number of questions you answer correctly, which is then converted into a scaled score, taking into account the difficulty of the test items. The passing score for each of the two exam sections is 75 (scaled). In order to pass the Board Exam, test-takers must achieve passing scores on *both* the Arts and Sciences sections. Those who fail one or both sections may retake the section(s) until they pass.

HOW TO TAKE A TEST

You have studied long, hard and conscientiously.

With your official admission card in hand, and your heart pounding, you have been admitted to the examination room.

You note that there are several hundred other applicants in the examination room waiting to take the same test.

They all appear to be equally well prepared.

You know that nothing but your best effort will suffice. The "moment of truth" is at hand: you now have to demonstrate objectively, in writing, your knowledge of content and your understanding of subject matter.

You are fighting the most important battle of your life—to pass and/or score high on an examination which will determine your career and provide the economic basis for your livelihood.

What extra, special things should you know and should you do in taking the examination?

I. YOU MUST PASS AN EXAMINATION

A. WHAT EVERY CANDIDATE SHOULD KNOW
Examination applicants often ask us for help in preparing for the written test. What can I study in advance? What kinds of questions will be asked? How will the test be given? How will the papers be graded?

B. HOW ARE EXAMS DEVELOPED?
Examinations are carefully written by trained technicians who are specialists in the field known as "psychological measurement," in consultation with recognized authorities in the field of work that the test will cover. These experts recommend the subject matter areas or skills to be tested; only those knowledges or skills important to your success on the job are included. The most reliable books and source materials available are used as references. Together, the experts and technicians judge the difficulty level of the questions.
Test technicians know how to phrase questions so that the problem is clearly stated. Their ethics do not permit "trick" or "catch" questions. Questions may have been tried out on sample groups, or subjected to statistical analysis, to determine their usefulness.
Written tests are often used in combination with performance tests, ratings of training and experience, and oral interviews. All of these measures combine to form the best-known means of finding the right person for the right job.

II. HOW TO PASS THE WRITTEN TEST

A. BASIC STEPS

1) Study the announcement

How, then, can you know what subjects to study? Our best answer is: "Learn as much as possible about the class of positions for which you've applied." The exam will test the knowledge, skills and abilities needed to do the work.

Your most valuable source of information about the position you want is the official exam announcement. This announcement lists the training and experience qualifications. Check these standards and apply only if you come reasonably close to meeting them. Many jurisdictions preview the written test in the exam announcement by including a section called "Knowledge and Abilities Required," "Scope of the Examination," or some similar heading. Here you will find out specifically what fields will be tested.

2) Choose appropriate study materials

If the position for which you are applying is technical or advanced, you will read more advanced, specialized material. If you are already familiar with the basic principles of your field, elementary textbooks would waste your time. Concentrate on advanced textbooks and technical periodicals. Think through the concepts and review difficult problems in your field.

These are all general sources. You can get more ideas on your own initiative, following these leads. For example, training manuals and publications of the government agency which employs workers in your field can be useful, particularly for technical and professional positions. A letter or visit to the government department involved may result in more specific study suggestions, and certainly will provide you with a more definite idea of the exact nature of the position you are seeking.

3) Study this book!

III. KINDS OF TESTS

Tests are used for purposes other than measuring knowledge and ability to perform specified duties. For some positions, it is equally important to test ability to make adjustments to new situations or to profit from training. In others, basic mental abilities not dependent on information are essential. Questions which test these things may not appear as pertinent to the duties of the position as those which test for knowledge and information. Yet they are often highly important parts of a fair examination. For very general questions, it is almost impossible to help you direct your study efforts. What we can do is to point out some of the more common of these general abilities needed in public service positions and describe some typical questions.

1) General information

Broad, general information has been found useful for predicting job success in some kinds of work. This is tested in a variety of ways, from vocabulary lists to questions about current events. Basic background in some field of work, such as sociology or economics, may be sampled in a group of questions. Often these are principles which have become familiar to most persons through exposure rather than through formal training. It is difficult to advise you how to study for these questions; being alert to the world around you is our best suggestion.

2) Verbal ability

An example of an ability needed in many positions is verbal or language ability. Verbal ability is, in brief, the ability to use and understand words. Vocabulary and grammar tests are typical measures of this ability. Reading comprehension or paragraph interpretation questions are common in many kinds of civil service tests. You are given a paragraph of written material and asked to find its central meaning.

IV. KINDS OF QUESTIONS

1. Multiple-choice Questions

Most popular of the short-answer questions is the "multiple choice" or "best answer" question. It can be used, for example, to test for factual knowledge, ability to solve problems or judgment in meeting situations found at work.

A multiple-choice question is normally one of three types:
- It can begin with an incomplete statement followed by several possible endings. You are to find the one ending which best completes the statement, although some of the others may not be entirely wrong.
- It can also be a complete statement in the form of a question which is answered by choosing one of the statements listed.
- It can be in the form of a problem – again you select the best answer.

Here is an example of a multiple-choice question with a discussion which should give you some clues as to the method for choosing the right answer:

When an employee has a complaint about his assignment, the action which will best help him overcome his difficulty is to
- A. discuss his difficulty with his coworkers
- B. take the problem to the head of the organization
- C. take the problem to the person who gave him the assignment
- D. say nothing to anyone about his complaint

In answering this question, you should study each of the choices to find which is best. Consider choice "A" – Certainly an employee may discuss his complaint with fellow employees, but no change or improvement can result, and the complaint remains unresolved. Choice "B" is a poor choice since the head of the organization probably does not know what assignment you have been given, and taking your problem to him is known as "going over the head" of the supervisor. The supervisor, or person who made the assignment, is the person who can clarify it or correct any injustice. Choice "C" is, therefore, correct. To say nothing, as in choice "D," is unwise. Supervisors have and interest in knowing the problems employees are facing, and the employee is seeking a solution to his problem.

2. True/False

3. Matching Questions

Matching an answer from a column of choices within another column.

V. RECORDING YOUR ANSWERS

Computer terminals are used more and more today for many different kinds of exams.

For an examination with very few applicants, you may be told to record your answers in the test booklet itself. Separate answer sheets are much more common. If this separate answer sheet is to be scored by machine – and this is often the case – it is highly important that you mark your answers correctly in order to get credit.

VI. BEFORE THE TEST

YOUR PHYSICAL CONDITION IS IMPORTANT

If you are not well, you can't do your best work on tests. If you are half asleep, you can't do your best either. Here are some tips:

1) Get about the same amount of sleep you usually get. Don't stay up all night before the test, either partying or worrying—DON'T DO IT!
2) If you wear glasses, be sure to wear them when you go to take the test. This goes for hearing aids, too.
3) If you have any physical problems that may keep you from doing your best, be sure to tell the person giving the test. If you are sick or in poor health, you relay cannot do your best on any test. You can always come back and take the test some other time.

Common sense will help you find procedures to follow to get ready for an examination. Too many of us, however, overlook these sensible measures. Indeed, nervousness and fatigue have been found to be the most serious reasons why applicants fail to do their best on civil service tests. Here is a list of reminders:

- Begin your preparation early – Don't wait until the last minute to go scurrying around for books and materials or to find out what the position is all about.
- Prepare continuously – An hour a night for a week is better than an all-night cram session. This has been definitely established. What is more, a night a week for a month will return better dividends than crowding your study into a shorter period of time.
- Locate the place of the exam – You have been sent a notice telling you when and where to report for the examination. If the location is in a different town or otherwise unfamiliar to you, it would be well to inquire the best route and learn something about the building.
- Relax the night before the test – Allow your mind to rest. Do not study at all that night. Plan some mild recreation or diversion; then go to bed early and get a good night's sleep.
- Get up early enough to make a leisurely trip to the place for the test – This way unforeseen events, traffic snarls, unfamiliar buildings, etc. will not upset you.
- Dress comfortably – A written test is not a fashion show. You will be known by number and not by name, so wear something comfortable.
- Leave excess paraphernalia at home – Shopping bags and odd bundles will get in your way. You need bring only the items mentioned in the official notice you received; usually everything you need is provided. Do not bring reference books to the exam. They will only confuse those last minutes and be taken away from you when in the test room.

- Arrive somewhat ahead of time – If because of transportation schedules you must get there very early, bring a newspaper or magazine to take your mind off yourself while waiting.
- Locate the examination room – When you have found the proper room, you will be directed to the seat or part of the room where you will sit. Sometimes you are given a sheet of instructions to read while you are waiting. Do not fill out any forms until you are told to do so; just read them and be prepared.
- Relax and prepare to listen to the instructions
- If you have any physical problem that may keep you from doing your best, be sure to tell the test administrator. If you are sick or in poor health, you really cannot do your best on the exam. You can come back and take the test some other time.

VII. AT THE TEST

The day of the test is here and you have the test booklet in your hand. The temptation to get going is very strong. Caution! There is more to success than knowing the right answers. You must know how to identify your papers and understand variations in the type of short-answer question used in this particular examination. Follow these suggestions for maximum results from your efforts:

1) Cooperate with the monitor

The test administrator has a duty to create a situation in which you can be as much at ease as possible. He will give instructions, tell you when to begin, check to see that you are marking your answer sheet correctly, and so on. He is not there to guard you, although he will see that your competitors do not take unfair advantage. He wants to help you do your best.

2) Listen to all instructions

Don't jump the gun! Wait until you understand all directions. In most civil service tests you get more time than you need to answer the questions. So don't be in a hurry. Read each word of instructions until you clearly understand the meaning. Study the examples, listen to all announcements and follow directions. Ask questions if you do not understand what to do.

3) Identify your papers

Civil service exams are usually identified by number only. You will be assigned a number; you must not put your name on your test papers. Be sure to copy your number correctly. Since more than one exam may be given, copy your exact examination title.

4) Plan your time

Unless you are told that a test is a "speed" or "rate of work" test, speed itself is usually not important. Time enough to answer all the questions will be provided, but this does not mean that you have all day. An overall time limit has been set. Divide the total time (in minutes) by the number of questions to determine the approximate time you have for each question.

5) Do not linger over difficult questions

If you come across a difficult question, mark it with a paper clip (useful to have along) and come back to it when you have been through the booklet. One caution if you do this – be sure to skip a number on your answer sheet as well. Check often to be sure that you have not lost your place and that you are marking in the row numbered the same as the question you are answering.

6) Read the questions

Be sure you know what the question asks! Many capable people are unsuccessful because they failed to read the questions correctly.

7) Answer all questions

Unless you have been instructed that a penalty will be deducted for incorrect answers, it is better to guess than to omit a question.

8) Speed tests

It is often better NOT to guess on speed tests. It has been found that on timed tests people are tempted to spend the last few seconds before time is called in marking answers at random – without even reading them – in the hope of picking up a few extra points. To discourage this practice, the instructions may warn you that your score will be "corrected" for guessing. That is, a penalty will be applied. The incorrect answers will be deducted from the correct ones, or some other penalty formula will be used.

9) Review your answers

If you finish before time is called, go back to the questions you guessed or omitted to give them further thought. Review other answers if you have time.

10) Return your test materials

If you are ready to leave before others have finished or time is called, take ALL your materials to the monitor and leave quietly. Never take any test material with you. The monitor can discover whose papers are not complete, and taking a test booklet may be grounds for disqualification.

VIII. EXAMINATION TECHNIQUES

1) Read the general instructions carefully. These are usually printed on the first page of the exam booklet. As a rule, these instructions refer to the timing of the examination; the fact that you should not start work until the signal and must stop work at a signal, etc. If there are any special instructions, such as a choice of questions to be answered, make sure that you note this instruction carefully.

2) When you are ready to start work on the examination, that is as soon as the signal has been given, read the instructions to each question booklet, underline any key words or phrases, such as least, best, outline, describe and the like. In this way you will tend to answer as requested rather than discover on reviewing your paper that you listed without describing, that you selected the worst choice rather than the best choice, etc.

3) If the examination is of the objective or multiple-choice type – that is, each question will also give a series of possible answers: A, B, C or D, and you are called upon to select the best answer and write the letter next to that answer on your answer paper – it is advisable to start answering each question in turn. There may be anywhere from 50 to 100 such questions in the three or four hours allotted and you can see how much time would be taken if you read through all the questions before beginning to answer any. Furthermore, if you

come across a question or group of questions which you know would be difficult to answer, it would undoubtedly affect your handling of all the other questions.

4) If the examination is of the essay type and contains but a few questions, it is a moot point as to whether you should read all the questions before starting to answer any one. Of course, if you are given a choice – say five out of seven and the like – then it is essential to read all the questions so you can eliminate the two that are most difficult. If, however, you are asked to answer all the questions, there may be danger in trying to answer the easiest one first because you may find that you will spend too much time on it. The best technique is to answer the first question, then proceed to the second, etc.

5) Time your answers. Before the exam begins, write down the time it started, then add the time allowed for the examination and write down the time it must be completed, then divide the time available somewhat as follows:
    - If 3-1/2 hours are allowed, that would be 210 minutes. If you have 80 objective-type questions, that would be an average of 2-1/2 minutes per question. Allow yourself no more than 2 minutes per question, or a total of 160 minutes, which will permit about 50 minutes to review.
    - If for the time allotment of 210 minutes there are 7 essay questions to answer, that would average about 30 minutes a question. Give yourself only 25 minutes per question so that you have about 35 minutes to review.

6) The most important instruction is to read each question and make sure you know what is wanted. The second most important instruction is to time yourself properly so that you answer every question. The third most important instruction is to answer every question. Guess if you have to but include something for each question. Remember that you will receive no credit for a blank and will probably receive some credit if you write something in answer to an essay question. If you guess a letter – say "B" for a multiple-choice question – you may have guessed right. If you leave a blank as an answer to a multiple-choice question, the examiners may respect your feelings but it will not add a point to your score. Some exams may penalize you for wrong answers, so in such cases only, you may not want to guess unless you have some basis for your answer.

7) Suggestions
    a. Objective-type questions
        1. Examine the question booklet for proper sequence of pages and questions
        2. Read all instructions carefully
        3. Skip any question which seems too difficult; return to it after all other questions have been answered
        4. Apportion your time properly; do not spend too much time on any single question or group of questions
        5. Note and underline key words – all, most, fewest, least, best, worst, same, opposite, etc.
        6. Pay particular attention to negatives
        7. Note unusual option, e.g., unduly long, short, complex, different or similar in content to the body of the question
        8. Observe the use of "hedging" words – probably, may, most likely, etc.

9. Make sure that your answer is put next to the same number as the question
10. Do not second-guess unless you have good reason to believe the second answer is definitely more correct
11. Cross out original answer if you decide another answer is more accurate; do not erase until you are ready to hand your paper in
12. Answer all questions; guess unless instructed otherwise
13. Leave time for review

b. Essay questions
   1. Read each question carefully
   2. Determine exactly what is wanted. Underline key words or phrases.
   3. Decide on outline or paragraph answer
   4. Include many different points and elements unless asked to develop any one or two points or elements
   5. Show impartiality by giving pros and cons unless directed to select one side only
   6. Make and write down any assumptions you find necessary to answer the questions
   7. Watch your English, grammar, punctuation and choice of words
   8. Time your answers; don't crowd material

8) Answering the essay question

Most essay questions can be answered by framing the specific response around several key words or ideas. Here are a few such key words or ideas:

M's: manpower, materials, methods, money, management
P's: purpose, program, policy, plan, procedure, practice, problems, pitfalls, personnel, public relations

a. Six basic steps in handling problems:
   1. Preliminary plan and background development
   2. Collect information, data and facts
   3. Analyze and interpret information, data and facts
   4. Analyze and develop solutions as well as make recommendations
   5. Prepare report and sell recommendations
   6. Install recommendations and follow up effectiveness

b. Pitfalls to avoid
1. Taking things for granted – A statement of the situation does not necessarily imply that each of the elements is necessarily true; for example, a complaint may be invalid and biased so that all that can be taken for granted is that a complaint has been registered
2. Considering only one side of a situation – Wherever possible, indicate several alternatives and then point out the reasons you selected the best one
3. Failing to indicate follow up – Whenever your answer indicates action on your part, make certain that you will take proper follow-up action to see how successful your recommendations, procedures or actions turn out to be
4. Taking too long in answering any single question – Remember to time your answers properly

EXAMINATION SECTION

EXAMINATION SECTION
TEST 1

DIRECTIONS: Each question or incomplete statement is followed by several suggested answers or completions. Select the one that BEST answers the question or completes the statement. *PRINT THE LETTER OF THE CORRECT ANSWER IN THE SPACE AT THE RIGHT.*

1. "High-index" embalming fluids are those that have a formaldehyde index of about   1._____

    A. 23 to 27
    B. 25 to 30
    C. 30 to 35
    D. 42 to 45

2. The Egyptians' elaborate precautions to preserve the remains of their dead stemmed from their belief that   2._____

    A. the wealth and well-being of survivors was linked to the intactness of their ancestor's bodies
    B. there would be a day when all the dead would rise up again and walk the earth
    C. decompositions was a kind of desecration
    D. the soul of the deceased remained in the mummified body

3. Which of the following items of information can be lawfully solicited from an applicant during an employment interview for the purpose of disqualification?   3._____

    A. Prior marital status
    B. Whether candidate has ever worked under a different name
    C. Military discharge status, if not the result of a military conviction
    D. Arrest record

4. When a preneed funeral contract is guaranteed, this means that the   4._____

    A. funeral home will provide the funeral services and merchandise selected at the cost of those items at the time of your funeral
    B. the
    C. price of the funeral services and merchandise will not exceed the balance in the trust account at the time the funeral is provided
    D. agreement may not be transferred to another funeral home

5. The embalming process typically takes from _____ hours.   5._____

    A. 1.5 to 2.5
    B. 3.5 to 5.5
    C. 6 to 8
    D. 24 to 48

6. According to Wolfelt, people who make an effort to "keep busy" after a loved one dies are most likely to   6._____

    A. temporarily distract themselves from their grief
    B. suffer a psychotic episode
    C. increase stress by postponing discussions of thoughts and feelings
    D. be able to forget about their loved ones for long periods of time

7. What is the legal term for the reversion of property to the state upon the death of the owner when there are no heirs?

   A. Intestate
   B. Probate
   C. Cloture
   D. Escheat

8. A casket is made of ferrous metal, 1/16-inch thick. This thickness corresponds to a gauge of

   A. 8
   B. 16
   C. 32
   D. 48

9. Formaldehyde solutions that are too harsh are MOST likely to produce a

   A. green discoloration
   B. jaundived appearance
   C. bleached white appearance
   D. graying of the tissues

10. The most common method for simulating pores involves a

    A. mild caustic solution
    B. small-bore hypodermic needle
    C. medium-nap roller
    D. stipple brush

11. Interior styles for caskets include each of the following, EXCEPT

    A. tufted
    B. crushed
    C. polished
    D. shirred

12. Of the following accounts, _____ normally has a credit balance.

    A. prepare expenses
    B. assets
    C. liabilities
    D. expenses

13. A family has purchased an oversize casket for their deceased relative. In the casket price list, the casket size is followed by the letters "XX." This casket is
    I. two inches wider than the average casket
    II. twice the size of the average casket
    III. six inches longer than the average casket
    IV. four inches wider than the average casket

    A. I only   B. II only   C. III and IV   D. IV only

14. It is generally recommended by practitioners in the helping professions that survivors of a traumatic event that resulted in the sudden death of others should   14._____

    A. avoid support groups and other settings that might invoke unpleasant memories
    B. talk about the event if the subject comes up
    C. avoid discussing the event, but think about it often
    D. treat the resulting pain and depression primarily with medications

15. The thoracic cavity is divided into two parts by the   15._____

    A. peritoneum
    B. mediastinum
    C. pleural cavity
    D. diaphragm

16. Which of the following is typically performed FIRST by a person who trains others in communication skills?   16._____

    A. Rehearsal
    B. Modeling
    C. Feedback
    D. Reinforcement

17. Which of the following is NOT a sign associated with impaired oxygen profusion?   17._____

    A. Bradycardia
    B. Diaphoresis
    C. Clammy skin
    D. Restlessness

18. Bacteria that die in the presence of oxygen are described as _____ anaerobes.   18._____

    A. nanaerobic
    B. obligate
    C. fermenting
    D. facultative

19. Over the past several decades, general trends among American families have included   19._____
    I. a rising average age for first marriages
    II. an increasing in the rate at which married women with children join the workforce
    III. more geographic stability, with fewer major moves
    IV. fewer single mothers than ever before

    A. I and II
    B. II and III
    C. II, III and IV
    D. I, II, III and IV

20. What is the term for blame that is perceived to be directed at oneself by others?   20._____

    A. Compunction
    B. Anger
    C. Shame
    D. Guilt

21. The chemical components of embalming fluid are suspended in a liquid medium known as a vehicle. Which of the following is NOT a common vehicle used in enbalming fluid?

   A. Methanol
   B. Phenol
   C. Water
   D. Glycerin

22. When all the parties interested in a joint contract die, an action must be brought by

   A. a covenantor against a survivor
   B. the executors or administrators of the last surviving obligor, against the executors or administrators of the last surviving obligee
   C. a survivor against a covenantor
   D. the executors or administrators of the last surviving obligee, against the executors or administrators of the last surviving obligor

23. A funeral director wishes to contract with a common carrier to transport the remains of a person who has died in another country. As a general rule, most common carriers require

   A. payment in advance
   B. that the body be prepared in a way that requires no special shipping circumstance
   C. the body to be embalmed before shipping
   D. the body to be cremated before shipping

24. The funeral service practitioner must constantly be on guard against the feeling that his or her own cultural responses and activities relative to the death of a loved one is superior to that of other cultures. Such a belief, whether conscious or not, is an example of

   A. cultural relativism
   B. an adaptive rite
   C. ethnocentrism
   D. a taboo

25. In _____ funerals, the casket of the deceased is reopened just before burial to allow loved ones to look at the deceased one last time and give their final farewells.

   A. Orthodox Jewish
   B. Roman Catholic
   C. Eastern Orthodox
   D. Orthodox Muslim

KEY (CORRECT ANSWERS)

1.	C	11.	C
2.	D	12.	B
3.	B	13.	C
4.	C	14.	B
5.	A	15.	B
6.	C	16.	B
7.	D	17.	A
8.	B	18.	B
9.	D	19.	A
10.	D	20.	C

21. B
22. D
23. C
24. C
25. C

TEST 2

DIRECTIONS: Each question or incomplete statement is followed by several suggested answers or completions. Select the one that BEST answers the question or completes the statement. *PRINT THE LETTER OF THE CORRECT ANSWER IN THE SPACE AT THE RIGHT.*

1. Liquid complexion cosmetics that are _____ can be applied satisfactorily onto restoration wax.

    A. suspensions
    B. water-based
    C. colloidal
    D. oil-based

2. In most jurisdictions, the cremation of a body immediately following death

    A. is generally permissible
    B. requires a legal waiver by a medical examiner or justice of the peace
    C. requires the signature of the next of kin
    D. is never permissible, under any circumstances

3. The _____ vein is classified as a deep vein.

    A. median cubital
    B. brachial
    C. great saphenous
    D. cephalic

4. What is the term for a structure or building designed for the housing of urns of cremsed remains in niches?

    A. Crypt
    B. Catacomb
    C. Columbarium
    D. Catafalque

5. The fourth stage of anticipatory grief, described by Kubler-Ross, is

    A. bargaining
    B. denial
    C. depression
    D. acceptance

6. The antibody produced FIRST during an infection is

    A. IgM
    B. IgG
    C. IgE
    D. IgA

7. Which of the following religious denominations is MOST likely to discourage eulogies at the funeral and burials services?

    A. Baptist
    B. Unitarian
    C. Methodist
    D. Roman Catholic

8. Surface gels used in embalming may contain _____ to facilitate the penetration of preservatives.

   A. sodium lauryl sulfate
   B. sodium citrate
   C. phenol
   D. carbolic acid

9. What is the term used to describe family members who appear to be over-involved or overprotective of another family member?

   A. Enmeshed
   B. Transferent
   C. Projective
   D. Dysfunctional

10. The most common malignant neoplasm involving the lung is

    A. hamartoma
    B. carcinoid tumor
    C. metastatic carcinoma
    D. bronchioloalveolar carcinoma

11. At its base, the nose is typically as wide as the

    A. mouth
    B. eye
    C. ear
    D. wrist

12. Input devices for a computer include the
    I. touch screen
    II. keyboard
    III. mouse
    IV. scanner

    A. I only
    B. I and IV
    C. II and III
    D. I, II, III and IV

13. The _____ vein drains blood from the posterior thoracic wall and delivers blood to the superior vena cava.

    A. azygos
    B. brachial
    C. cephalic
    D. basilir

14. _____ are instruments drawn in special form that can be transferred from person to person as a substitute for money, or as an instrument of credit.

    A. Liquidities
    B. Negotiable instruments
    C. Certificates of deposit
    D. Commodities

15. The term _____ damages refers to the reasonable estimate of the damages that would result from a contractual breach by the parties, and is stipulated in the contract.

    A. liquidated
    B. mitigated
    C. cancelled
    D. executory

16. A decedent was not married and had no children, but she left a valid will. Each of the following would have a right to final disposition, EXCEPT

    A. a sibling
    B. a parent
    C. a personal representative of the estate
    D. the state

17. Factors used to determine the strength and amount of embalming fluid to use on a given case include
    I. time between death and preparation
    II. weight of the body
    III. amount of adipose tissue vs. muscular tissue
    IV. protein levels in the body

    A. I only
    B. II only
    C. I, II and III
    D. I, II, III and IV

18. Friends or family members who are designated as "honorary pallbearers" typically

    A. escort individual mourners into the church or building where the funeral sendee is held
    B. carry the casket to and from the funeral service
    C. act as an escort or honor guard for the deceased
    D. have their names included on the program, but do not participate in the sendee

19. Funeral claims against the estate of the deceased are considered to be

    A. in the same category as any other debt
    B. secondary to most other forms of debt
    C. preferred claims
    D. illegal when filed

20. _____ is the term used to describe the process of transferring entries from a company's journals to its ledger accounts.

    A. Posting
    B. Double-entry
    C. Reconciliation
    D. Cross-footing

21. Of the following religious groups, which prohibit the practice of cremation?

    I. Buddhists
    II. Roman Catholics
    III. Orthodox Jews
    IV. Muslims

    A. I and IV
    B. II and III
    C. III and IV
    D. I, II, III and IV

22. To close incisions made for the purpose of embalming, most practitioners use a suture known as the _____ stitch.

    A. whip
    B. double intradermal
    C. N
    D. baseball

23. In Celtic tribal societies, the dead were placed near villages in groups of graves that were covered by raised mounds known as

    A. wights
    B. middens
    C. stelae
    D. barrows

24. Which of the following will result when discounts, sales returns, and allowances are subtracted from gross sales?

    A. Gross profit
    B. Net sales
    C. Total purchases
    D. Current inventory

25. Under OSHA's _____ standards, funeral homes are required to provide specific training, protective clothing, and a vaccination against hepatitis B.

    A. Bloodborne Pathogens
    B. Means of Egress
    C. Respiratory Protection
    D. Hazard Communication

KEY (CORRECT ANSWERS)

1. C
2. B
3. B
4. C
5. C

6. A
7. D
8. A
9. A
10. C

11. B
12. D
13. A
14. B
15. A

16. D
17. D
18. C
19. C
20. A

21. C
22. D
23. D
24. B
25. A

TEST 3

DIRECTIONS: Each question or incomplete statement is followed by several suggested answers or completions. Select the one that BEST answers the question or completes the statement. *PRINT THE LETTER OF THE CORRECT ANSWER IN THE SPACE AT THE RIGHT.*

1. A restorer making an incision often chooses to undercut, rather than cut perpendicularly. The undercut involves each of the following advantages, EXCEPT

    A. no need to extend wax far beyond margins
    B. no need to trim off hard, dehydrated tissue at the margin
    C. undercut edge helps lock wax in position
    D. no need for a basket-weave suture

    1._____

2. An irrevocable preneed funeral contract typically specifies that

    A. the funeral home must limit its services to the funds available in the trust
    B. excess funds cannot be refunded if the amount in the trust account is less than the cost of the funeral
    C. the agreement may not be transferred to another funeral home
    D. services and merchandise cannot be changed after the agreement is made

    2._____

3. Which of the following customs or traditions is MOST likely to be involved in an orthodox Jewish funeral?

    A. Flowers placed over the grave of the deceased
    B. A plain wooden casket with no metal parts or adornments
    C. Cremation
    D. An avoidance of speaking of the deceased

    3._____

4. Chronic alcoholics often exhibit cardiac dilation, sight loss, peripheral neuropathy, muscle wasting, and generalized edema, all signs that are characteristic of

    A. iron deficiency
    B. Vitamin D deficiency
    C. cachexia
    D. Vitamin B1 deficiency

    4._____

5. The movement of gases within the body by applying external pressure is called

    A. translocation
    B. crepitation
    C. palpation
    D. auscultation

    5._____

6. Which of the following is NOT an advantage associated with a sole proprietorship?

    A. Profit incentive
    B. Freedom to manage
    C. Limited risk
    D. Low cost of organization

    6._____

7. Each of the following is a paranasal sinus, EXCEPT the _____ sinus.

    A. mastoid
    B. maxillary
    C. frontal
    D. ethmoidal

    7._____

8. _____ is a term applicable to the difference between expenses and revenue, assuming revenues are greater.

   A. Net profit
   B. Net worth
   C. Gross sales
   D. Gross margin

9. A _____ is typically required by the Veterans Administration in order for a deceased person to obtain federal burial benefits.

   A. separation/discharge form
   B. birth certificate
   C. Selective Service number
   D. Social Security number

10. Jaundice fluid typically has

    A. no coulter-staining effect
    B. no bleach content
    C. a low formaldehyde content
    D. a high formaldehyde content

11. Which of the following terms best describes a helping relationship in which one person seeks to facilitate the development of informed choices and meaningful actions at a critical time in another person's life?

    A. Counseling
    B. Psychotherapy
    C. Crisis intervention
    D. Companionship

12. Most jurisdictions, when a death occurs, require
    I. local law enforcement to be contacted if the death was unattended
    II. a determination of death by a coroner, attending physician, or justice of the peace
    III. funeral service practitioners to refrain from solicitation at or near the time of death
    IV. embalming or disposition within 48 hours

    A. I only
    B. I, II and III
    C. II only
    D. I, II, III and IV

13. In a(n) _____ contract, either party's performance is dependent on an uncertain event.

    A. verbal
    B. aleatory
    C. bonded
    D. accessory

14. The hairs of the eyebrow typically grow

    A. up and outward
    B. up and inward
    C. down and outward
    D. down and inward

15. A circumstance that divests contractual liability that has already attached upon the failure of the other party to comply with its terms is a

    A. frustration of purpose
    B. condition precedent
    C. consequential damage
    D. condition subsequent

16. Which of the following does Wolfelt identify as characteristic of stress?

    A. Impatience and irritability
    B. Increased creativity
    C. Impaired speech
    D. Focused concentration

17. To most families, the funeral rite
    I. serves to intensify grief to an unsustainable "breaking" point
    II. confirms the reality of death
    III. provides structure and activity for the bereaved
    IV. is a complex social event that serves to delay the full grieving process

    A. I and II
    B. II and III
    C. III only
    D. I, II, III and IV

18. Typically, the defense mechanism used to disguise anger that is easiest for other people to detect is

    A. weeping
    B. passive-aggressive behavior
    C. a self-righteousness attitude
    D. an over-reliance on reason

19. Although there is some difference of opinion on the number of caskets to have in a display room, it is generally considered that _____ is the minimum number of caskets that should be displayed, with _____ square feet allotted per casket.

    A. 5; 20 to 30
    B. 12; 40 to 60
    C. 20; 50 to 60
    D. 32; 65 to 80

20. The most basic factor that should be used to determine the beginning dilution of arterial embalming fluid is the   20._____

    A. condition of the body
    B. reaction produced by the chemicals injected
    C. size of the body
    D. cause of death

21. The _____ ledger contains all of the accounts shown on the trial balance.   21._____

    A. subsidiary
    B. accounts receivable
    C. audit
    D. general

22. The femoral artery is located in an area of the upper thigh known as   22._____

    A. Revinski's circle
    B. the Circle of Willis
    C. Clarke's column
    D. Scarpa's Triangle

23. What is the term for an amendment that changes the original provisions of a will?   23._____

    A. contest
    B. probate
    C. codicil
    D. testament

24. Which layer of the skin lies just above the fascia of the underlying muscle?   24._____

    A. Papillary layer
    B. Subcutaneous
    C. Sebaceous
    D. Dermis

25. Traditional Chinese funeral rites and burial customs were—and in many places still are—determined to a degree by the   25._____
    I. manner of the deceased's death
    II. age of the deceased
    III. deceased's social status
    IV. available burial space

    A. I only
    B. I, II and III
    C. II and III
    D. III and IV only

KEY (CORRECT ANSWERS)

1. B
2. B
3. B
4. D
5. B

6. C
7. A
8. A
9. A
10. C

11. A
12. B
13. B
14. A
15. D

16. A
17. B
18. B
19. B
20. A

21. D
22. D
23. C
24. B
25. B

TEST 4

DIRECTIONS: Each question or incomplete statement is followed by several suggested answers or completions. Select the one that BEST answers the question or completes the statement. *PRINT THE LETTER OF THE CORRECT ANSWER IN THE SPACE AT THE RIGHT.*

1. The reduction in body temperature following death is known as _____ _____ mortis.

    A. rigor
    B. algor
    C. pallor
    D. livor

    1._____

2. Chemicals that destroy the unpleasant odors of preservatives and disinfectants found in arterial fluid by chemically reacting with the source of the odor are

    A. surfactants
    B. humectants
    C. reodorants
    D. deodorants

    2._____

3. In the _____ selection room approach, the funeral director typically offers the highest level of support to the family.

    A. indirect
    B. direct
    C. hard-sell
    D. interpersonal

    3._____

4. Each of the following arteries supplies blood to the brain, EXCEPT the

    A. maxillary
    B. internal carotid
    C. external carotid
    D. basilar

    4._____

5. Diminished clotting factor activity is characteristic of

    A. kwashiorkor
    B. cachexia
    C. Vitamin K deficiency
    D. Vitamin B1 deficiency

    5._____

6. After the parents of a child have made their first viewing of a deceased family member in the funeral home, they approach the funeral service practitioner with their concerns about whether their 8-year-old child should also view the deceased. The practitioner should advise them that the child

    A. probably doesn't understand the reality of death, and a viewing is likely to be unimportant
    B. should view the deceased when the room contains as many other mourners as possible
    C. would most likely be too traumatized to benefit from a viewing
    D. should be encouraged, but not forced, to say a final goodbye

    6._____

7. The outer layer of the bone that serves as an attachment point for tendons and ligaments is the

   A. osteoblast
   B. periosteum
   C. fibrous layer
   D. epiphysis

8. The Fair Labor Standards Act covers each of the following areas of employment law, EXCEPT

   A. equal pay
   B. minimum age requirements for employment
   C. minimum wage requirements
   D. overtime compensation

9. Most likely, the custom of churchyard burial was begun by the _____, who wanted to have the bodies of those in their community as close to them as possible.

   A. Mesopotamians
   B. Ancient Greeks
   C. Christian monastic orders
   D. Egyptians

10. The _____ artery is the one most commonly used in the embalming process.

    A. femoral
    B. subclavian
    C. axillary
    D. carotid

11. Which of the following causes of death, stated on a death certificate, indicates a failure of the heart?

    A. Cerebrovascular accident
    B. Asphyxiation
    C. Myocardial infarction
    D. Pulmonary insufficiency

12. The lungs are _____ in relation to the heart.

    A. inferior
    B. superior
    C. medial
    D. lateral

13. Each of the following is an item required to be on the General Price List, EXCEPT

    A. alternative containers for direct cremation
    B. the Casket Price List
    C. use of automotive equipment for transport
    D. Basic Services Fee

14. Bowlby divided attachment theory into four phases. Which of the following was NOT one of them?

    A. Forming reciprocal relations with people
    B. Reacting with signals and behaviors toward any one person
    C. Reacting indiscriminately toward all people within a certain proximity
    D. Maintaining a proximity to a specific person through movement and signals

15. An en. balming practitioner wants to make one gallon of 2% fluid. About how many ounces of 25-index fluid will be needed?

    A. 10
    B. 12
    C. 18
    D. 25

16. Which of the following is NOT a symptom of grief, according to Lindemann?

    A. Preoccupation with the deceased
    B. Clinical depression
    C. Shortness of breath
    D. Muscular weakness

17. A funeral service, held in a liturgical church, involves a processional and recessional that includes clergy, casket bearers, the casket of the deceased, and family. The aisle is not wide enough to accommodate both the casket and the casket bearers. During the processional and recessional, the casket bearers should

    A. seat themselves in the last row of the church
    B. walk between the casket and the family
    C. walk in front of the casket, behind the clergy
    D. remain standing at the rear of the church

18. The record of a company's liabilities, assets, and owner's equity can be found on the

    A. journal
    B. balance sheet
    C. income statement
    D. trial balance

19. A person who is able to make him or herself independent from others by means of separating the intellect from the emotions is said to have achieved

    A. differentiation
    B. a psychotic break
    C. socialization
    D. Nirvana

20. When using hypodermic tissue builder, the restorer/enbalmer should

    A. use tissue builder solvent is a dissolving agent if too much builder is injected in the tissues
    B. clean the needle and syringe with water
    C. inject slightly more than is needed and aspirate the excess later
    D. use a 17 gauge needle, or slightly smaller

21. The Sikh culture's view of death and funeral customs includes each of the following, EXCEPT a belief that

    A. burial is the preferred method of disposal
    B. the human soul is reincarnated
    C. permanent commemoration with gravestones is discouraged
    D. public displays of grief at the funeral service should be kept to a minimum

22. The most common cause of death that occurs within the first two hours following an acute myocardial infarction is

    A. arrhythmia
    B. loss of myosin from injured cells
    C. myocardial rupture
    D. loss of calcium from sarcoplasmic reticulum

23. When a death is due to AIDS, the Americans with Disabilities Act (ADA) provides that a funeral home may
    I. insist on cremation
    II. charge more for embalming
    III. have a private service
    IV. require a sealed casket

    A. I only
    B. I and II
    C. III only
    D. II and IV

24. In a business ledger, a credit to accounts payable would have a corresponding debit to

    A. accounts receivable
    B. purchases
    C. sales expense
    D. inventory

25. In a procedure known as _____, an adult may restate his or her willingness to be bound *by a* promise made during an age of minority.

    A. rescindment
    B. exploitation
    C. *in media res*
    D. ratification

KEY (CORRECT ANSWERS)

1. B
2. D
3. B
4. A
5. C

6. D
7. B
8. A
9. C
10. D

11. C
12. D
13. C
14. C
15. A

16. B
17. C
18. B
19. A
20. D

21. A
22. A
23. C
24. B
25. D

TEST 5

DIRECTIONS: Each question or incomplete statement is followed by several suggested answers or completions. Select the one that BEST answers the question or completes the statement. *PRINT THE LETTER OF THE CORRECT ANSWER IN THE SPACE AT THE RIGHT.*

1. During a planning meeting, a customer reads the following message on a document: "You may choose only the items you desire. If you are charged for items that you did not specifically request, we will explain the reason for the charges on the written memorandum. Please note that there may be charges for items such as cemetery fees, flowers and newspaper notices."
 This notice is required by law to be printed on the

    A. General Price List
    B. Preneed contract
    C. Outer Burial Container Price List
    D. Casket Price List

2. With regard to funeral service, studies have shown that "baby boomers"
    I. are averse to caskets
    II. tend to opt for low-cost alternatives
    III. have weaker church ties than their parents
    IV. prefer services to focus on the celebration of life

    A. I and II
    B. I, III and IV
    C. II and IV
    D. I, II, III and IV

3. In ancient Rome, the burial of a paupers would most likely have been performed by a person known as a

    A. columbarium
    B. praeco
    C. libitinarius
    D. vespillo

4. "Opening and Closing" fees are charged by a

    A. funeral home, for initiating and concluding funeral services
    B. crematory, for cremating a body and sealing the remains in an urn or other container
    C. a cemetery, for the digging and refilling of a grave
    D. medical examiner, for initiating and concluding an inquiry into the cause of death

5. Mild embalming solutions (those with a lower formaldehyde index) are most typically used in cases where the deceased

    A. has been autopsied and refrigerated for more than 12 hours
    B. is emaciated
    C. has been frozen
    D. exhibits postmortem staining

6. Though a universal definition of "religion" is difficult to come by, it is widely recognized to include
   I. a system of beliefs
   II. a sense of meaning or relevance in relation to something greater than oneself
   III. customs and rituals associated with beliefs
   IV. an intellectual rather then emotional response to certain beliefs

   A. I only
   B. I and II
   C. I, II and III
   D. I, II, III and IV

   6.____

7. A person to whom a right or property is transferred under a contract is known as the

   A. obligor
   B. agent
   C. assignee
   D. assignor

   7.____

8. What is the term for the deduction of certain capital expenses over a fixed period of time?

   A. Income adjustment
   B. Amortization
   C. Itemization
   D. Adjusted basis

   8.____

9. Conditions that may result in an immunocompromised host include
   I. diabetes
   II. cancer
   III. alcoholism
   IV. malnutrition

   A. I only
   B. I and II
   C. II, III and IV
   D. I, II, III and IV

   9.____

10. If a funeral service practitioner intentionally misrepresents a benefit of a preneed funeral contract, _____ has occurred.

    A. misfeasance
    B. malice
    C. fraud
    D. duress

    10.____

11. During an employment interview, the solicitation of information about _____, in ANY situation, no matter what the perceived relationship to the job, is unlawful.
    I. race or color
    II. religion
    III. national origin
    IV. disabilities or handicaps

    A. I only   B. I and II   C. I, II and III   D. I, II, III and IV

    11.____

12. In a contract, the "consideration" offered could include each of the following, EXCEPT   12.____

    A. personal property
    B. money
    C. a promise to abstain from doing something illegal
    D. a promise to perform certain services

13. The most frequent cause of death from burns is   13.____

    A. fluid loss
    B. bacterial sepsis
    C. pulmonary damage
    D. neurogenic shock

14. OSHA rules require that medical records for each employee be preserved and maintained for a period that includes the duration of employment, plus an additional _____ years.   14.____

    A. 5
    B. 10
    C. 20
    D. 30

15. In determining whether a case has been properly embalmed, it is appropriate for the embalming practitioner to observe and determine each of the following, EXCEPT   15.____

    A. a change in the deceased's coloring
    B. the distention of veins
    C. the amount of time spent on the process
    D. a finning of the tissues

16. A(n)_____ is a legal instrument authorizing the payment of insurance benefits for funeral expenses to a funeral home.   16.____

    A. conveyance
    B. statement of insurability
    C. fiduciary bond
    D. assignment of proceeds

17. Objectives of pre-embalming restorations typically include   17.____

    I. alignment of torn tissues and deep cuts
    II. removal of loose or torn epidermis
    III. restoring contours of emaciated facial features
    IV. drainage of skin eruptions

    A. I, II and IV
    B. II, III and IV
    C. III only
    D. I, II, III and IV

18. A child at a funeral is fearful of approaching the casket, saying that the deceased might jump out at her. According to Grollman's conception of children's understanding of death, this child is most likely _____ years of age.

    A. 1-4
    B. 5-9
    C. 10-14
    D. 15-19

19. When the dermis has been exposed to air it often turns hard and brown, and should be restored in the same manner as a(n)

    A. abrasion
    B. tumor
    C. puncture
    D. mold or fungal infection

20. The preservative action of formaldehyde works by cross-linking _____ atoms.

    A. carbon
    B. hydrogen
    C. nitrogen
    D. oxygen

21. Compared to a 24-gauge steel casket, a 12-gauge steel casket would be

    A. the same thickness, but a different density
    B. thicker, but with less tensile strength
    C. thinner and lighter
    D. thicker and heavier

22. At the height of ancient Greek civilization, most Athenian graves were

    A. marked with inscribed stone tablets
    B. marked with a simple wooden plaque that decomposed quickly
    C. gathered together in vast underground catacombs
    D. unmarked plots in areas of mass burial

23. In severely disturbed families, separation and loss are most likely to be dealt with by

    A. indulging in fantasy and denial
    B. extending identities beyond the family
    C. exhibiting psychotic or self-destructive behaviors
    D. introducing an entirely new family dynamic

24. The intent of the funeral rite is to
    I. provide a forum for the gathering of the deceased's loved ones
    II. allow family and friends to summon their faith and beliefs concerning death
    III. honor the life of the deceased
    IV. complete the grieving process

    A. I only
    B. I, II and III
    C. II and III
    D. I, II, III and IV

25. An increasing trend in funeral services, at least in the United States, is the 25._____
    A. hosting of services at home, rather than in a church
    B. insistence on burial in religious churchyards or cemeteries
    C. burial of the deceased with several of his or her most prized material possessions
    D. proliferation of less formal memorial sendees

KEY (CORRECT ANSWERS)

1.	A	11.	A
2.	B	12.	C
3.	D	13.	B
4.	C	14.	D
5.	B	15.	C
6.	C	16.	D
7.	C	17.	A
8.	B	18.	A
9.	D	19.	A
10.	C	20.	C

21. D
22. A
23. A
24. B
25. D

EXAMINATION SECTION
TEST 1

DIRECTIONS: Each question or incomplete statement is followed by several suggested answers or completions. Select the one that BEST answers the question or completes the statement. *PRINT THE LETTER OF THE CORRECT ANSWER IN THE SPACE AT THE RIGHT.*

1. Normally, the greatest projection of the chin appears just

    A. above the labiomental sulcus
    B. below the labiomental sulcus
    C. below the lower lip
    D. below the platysmal sulci

    1.____

2. For a bacterial pathogen to be successful in growth and reproduction, it must find appropriate
    I. pH
    II. nutrients
    III. redox potential
    IV. temperature

    A. I and IV
    B. II, III and IV
    C. II and IV
    D. I, II, III and IV

    2.____

3. The primary purpose of intradermal sutures is to

    A. form a mesh to anchor wax
    B. hold the margins of incisions together
    C. correct distortion from sagging muscles
    D. temporarily hold retracted surface tissues in position

    3.____

4. A double-reinforced vault typically consists of a concrete layer plus a special-purpose liner made from

    A. epoxy
    B. latex
    C. stainless steel
    D. polyurethane

    4.____

5. On a death certificate, the "registrant" typically refers to the

    A. name of the deceased
    B. parent or guardian of the deceased
    C. informant or person who made the legal pronouncement of death
    D. person requesting certified copies of the death certificate

    5.____

6. A multipoint injection is usually required in the embalming process if
   I. death occurred within the previous 8 hours
   II. a one-point injection has been used but distribution cannot be observed
   III. death was caused by a ruptured aortic aneurysm
   IV. facial distention is anticipated

   A. I only
   B. II and III
   C. II, III and IV
   D. I, II, III and IV

7. During a funeral service at Pine Ridge Reservation, the body of a deceased member of a Lakota Sioux is placed on a burial scaffold. This kind of services would be called a(n)

   A. primitive ritual
   B. orthodoxy
   C. adaptive rite
   D. humanistic ceremony

8. The coronary arteries

   A. form the first arterial branch from the base of the aorta
   B. dilate and contract in rhythm with the heart ventricles
   C. supply part of the heart muscle with oxygen
   D. branch from the pulmonary veins

9. What is the legal term for the refusal to fulfill a voidable contract?

   A. Disavowal
   B. Negation
   C. Disaffirmance
   D. Repudiation

10. The most important sociological function of religion is to

    A. help divert people's attention from political or economic concerns
    B. decrease social stratification
    C. create meaning for people
    D. integrate people into society

11. A funeral director my legally discuss information on a death certificate with
    I. immediate family members of the deceased
    II. close friends of the deceased
    III. interested law enforcement officials
    IV. credentialed members of the news media

    A. I only
    B. I and III
    C. I, II and III
    D. I, II, III and IV

12. The primary function of word processing software is to

A. store data in a file
B. produce graphic presentations
C. list, calculate, and sort data
D. produce written documents

13. The external iliac artery lies along the medial border of the

    A. external oblique
    B. intercostals
    C. psoas major
    D. gastrocnemius

14. A funeral service practitioner is using the direct selection room procedure in helping a family select a vault. Under this procedure, the practitioner will

    A. refer the family the available vault catalogs, and then leave them alone
    B. refer the family the vault manufacturer
    C. leave the family to make their decision alone in the selection room
    D. remain with the family in the selection room

15. The _____ is the device used to evacuate fluids and gases from the abdominal and thoracic cavities.

    A. aneurism needle
    B. aspirator
    C. shunt
    D. trocar

16. What is the name traditionally given to a symbolic cloth covering place over the casket?

    A. Shroud
    B. Pall
    C. Veil
    D. Crepe

17. Most funeral service customers who opt for cremation prefer to dispose of the remains by

    A. burying them in the ground
    B. scattering them
    C. keeping them at home
    D. placing them in a niche

18. Ancient Roman funeral customs included each of the following, EXCEPT

    A. a feast held nine days after the disposal of the body
    B. a public procession to the tomb or pyre where the body was to be cremated
    C. poorer citizens buried by benevolent funerary societies
    D. cremation or burial within city limits

19. An embalmer should avoid using extremely hard water to dilute embalming fluid, because it can

A. stain tissues a gray color
B. prevent the fluid from permeating into the capillary space
C. coagulate the blood that remains in tissues
D. calcify just beneath the epidermi

20. Which of the following is NOT a maladaptive defense to against stress? 20.____

    A. Stereotyped patterns of behavior
    B. Reality-oriented solutions
    C. Unconscious reactions
    D. Fenerally passive reactions

21. A contract in which promises have not been fully performed by all parties is described as 21.____

    A. open
    B. executory
    C. voidable
    D. unexecuted

22. Each of the following is a business advantage associated with partnerships, EXCEPT 22.____

    A. combined talent and capital
    B. efficiency of labor
    C. ease of forming
    D. liquidity of investments

23. When a person has died from uremia, formaldehyde is likely to react with ammonia and produce 23.____

    A. the byproduct of water
    B. skin slippage
    C. gas bloat
    D. a sulfurous odor

24. As a general rule, the casket display room should 24.____
    I. be located on the main floor of the funeral home
    II. be in a separate building from the funeral home
    III. consist of several small rooms
    IV. consist of on large room

    A. I and III
    B. I and IV
    C. II and III
    D. II and IV

25. Each of the following is an appropriate use of *cavity* fluid, EXCEPT 25.____

    A. surface preservation of fetal remains
    B. drying and deodorizing surface lesions
    C. lending a more natural color to tissues
    D. preservation of viscera removed at autopsy

KEY (CORRECT ANSWERS)

1. B
2. D
3. B
4. D
5. A

6. B
7. C
8. A
9. C
10. D

11. B
12. D
13. C
14. D
15. D

16. B
17. B
18. D
19. C
20. B

21. B
22. D
23. A
24. B
25. C

TEST 2

DIRECTIONS: Each question or incomplete statement is followed by several suggested answers or completions. Select the one that BEST answers the question or completes the statement. *PRINT THE LETTER OF THE CORRECT ANSWER IN THE SPACE AT THE RIGHT.*

1. A customer and a funeral director have completed funeral arrangements. Under federal law, the purchase agreement that is given to the customer MUST
    I. be signed by the funeral director who assisted the customer
    II. lists the items selected from the General Price List
    III. list the cost of each item on the General Price List
    IV. contain an "escape clause" for both parties

    A. I and II
    B. I, II and III
    C. II and III only
    D. I, II, III and IV

2. In ancient Greece, it was customary to bury the dead

    A. outside religious temples
    B. on any ground that had first been consecrated by a priest
    C. along roadways or other areas outside the walls of towns
    D. in the private yards of individual homes

3. OSHA rules require that any work-related accident that results in a fatality be reported within _____ hours.

    A. 2
    B. 8
    C. 24
    D. 48

4. Socialization can be described as each of the following, EXCEPT

    A. the development of an individual personality
    B. a process of internalizing social values
    C. a perfect adjustment of the individual to societal demands
    D. a mutual process

5. Restorative treatments performed during arterial injection are usually designed to do each of the following, EXCEPT

    A. establish even preservation of face and hand tissues
    B. control swelling of facial tissues
    C. surface sanitizing of the body and external orifices
    D. bleach and lighten blood discolorations

6. The doctrine of the Roman Catholic Church specifies that cremated remains may be
    I. buried
    II. entombed
    III. scattered
    IV. kept at home

A. I only
B. I or II
C. I, II or III
D. I, II, III and IV

7. A(n) _____ preneed contract may be terminated by the purchaser at any time before the death of the beneficiary, with a refund of the money paid as prescribed by state law.

   A. revocable
   B. irrevocable
   C. non-guaranteed
   D. warrantable

8. Which of the following is a malignant neoplasm of the liver?

   A. cholangioma
   B. hamartoma
   C. adenoma
   D. adenocarcinoma

9. A quartet performing a funeral piece at the graveside is an example of a

   A. folkway
   B. custom
   C. rite
   D. ceremony

10. When used between applications of phenol solution, _____ can help halt the corrosive action.

    A. cavity fluid
    B. cyanoacrylate
    C. alcohol
    D. acetone

11. During the early medieval European period known as the Dark Ages, Christian burials in a church cemetery were denied to

    A. Celts
    B. divorcees
    C. plague victims
    D. suicides

12. The decompositions of proteins is known specifically as

    A. gangrene
    B. caries
    C. necrosis
    D. putrefaction

13. A humanistic service is one that

A. has no religious connotation
B. is considered a non-denominational Christian service
C. is held in a setting other than a place of worship
D. involves Masonic rites

14. What is the term for a contract cancellation that returns the parties to the positions they were in before the contract was made?

    A. Nullification
    B. Discharge
    C. Repudiation
    D. Rescission

15. Under the accrual method of accounting, business expenses are deductible during the year in which

    A. liability for payment is fixed
    B. goods are sold
    C. payment is actually made
    D. the payee includes the payment in income

16. A typical eight-year-old whose parent has just died is most likely to
    I. fail to mourn adequately
    II. believe death is a person or creature who has taken the parent away
    III. accept that death is final and inevitable
    IV. have no comprehension of death

    A. I and IV
    B. II and III
    C. I only
    D. III only

17. In the embalming process, the most common vein used for drainage is the

    A. subclavian
    B. femoral
    C. axillary
    D. jugular

18. Which of the following is another term for a church vestibule?

    A. Cupola
    B. Apse
    C. Narthex
    D. Chancel

19. The most reliable sign of arterial fluid distribution and diffusion is the

    A. presence of an active fluid dye in the tissues of the skin
    B. mottling of tissues
    C. drying of surface tissues
    D. loss of skin elasticity

20. People tend to pay attention to those features of their environment that are consistent with or reinforce their own expectations. This phenomenon is known as   20.____

    A. selective perception
    B. the Hawthorne effect
    C. ethnocentrism
    D. individualization

21. A funeral home uses the graduated recovery model for pricing its merchandise. The main advantage associated with this approach is that it   21.____

    A. provides a higher margin at the lower end
    B. makes lower-cost funerals available to lower-income customers
    C. provides good value at all points along the pricing spectrum
    D. applies positive pressure on the inventory

22. Mr. Mann was engaged by Rose Mortuary to paint the exterior of each of the buildings on the grounds. Mr. Mann was to be paid $4500, and the job was to completed within two weeks. Rose Mortuary was to have no control over how the painting was performed. Mr. Mann is considered a(n)   22.____

    A. agent of Rose Mortuary
    B. independent contractor
    C. vendor
    D. employee of Rose Mortuary

23. An employee has requested medical leave. Under federal employment law, the employer may require   23.____

    A. a statement from the employee's supervisor that he or she is unable to work
    B. a certificate from a healthcare provider attesting to the need for leave
    C. undeniable symptoms of illness or injury
    D. a previous history of illness or disease

24. _____ changes in a contract are those that extend the original scope of the agreement.   24.____

    A. constructive
    B. formal
    C. reconstructive
    D. cardinol

25. OSHA Standards include   25.____
    I. Machine Guarding
    II. Formaldehyde Exposure
    III. General Electrical
    IV. Hazard Communication

    A. I and II
    B. II and III
    C. III and IV
    D. I, II, III and IV

KEY (CORRECT ANSWERS)

1. B
2. C
3. B
4. C
5. C

6. B
7. A
8. A
9. D
10. C

11. D
12. D
13. A
14. D
15. A

16. B
17. D
18. C
19. A
20. A

21. B
22. B
23. B
24. D
25. D

TEST 3

DIRECTIONS: Each question or incomplete statement is followed by several suggested answers or completions. Select the one that BEST answers the question or completes the statement. *PRINT THE LETTER OF THE CORRECT ANSWER IN THE SPACE AT THE RIGHT.*

1. The word "cemetery" is formed from ancient Greek and Latin roots that can most closely be translated as

    A. final place
    B. great sorrow
    C. sleeping place
    D. unclean

    1.____

2. The final stage of Elisabeth Kubler-Ross's theory of how people handle the knowledge of impending death is

    A. acceptance
    B. anger
    C. bargaining
    D. denial

    2.____

3. A general partnership is typically characterized by each of the following, EXCEPT

    A. profit-sharing
    B. termination upon the death, disability, or withdrawal of any one partner
    C. transferable interest
    D. limited personal liability for losses

    3.____

4. Funeral service practitioners attempt to open the arrangement conference with a question that will put the family at ease and relieve some of their tensions. Which of the following would NOT be an appropriate question for this purpose?

    A. What are your thoughts on embalming?
    B. I didn't know your mother-could you tell me a little about her?
    C. Were you with your father when he died?
    D. What can we do together to plan the kind of funeral your brother would have wanted?

    4.____

5. In the embalming process, preinjection fluid
    I. contains a high level of preservative
    II. clears intravascular blood discolorations
    III. adjusts the pH of the tissues
    IV. removes blood from the vascular system

    A. I and II
    B. II and IV
    C. II, III and IV
    D. I, II, III and IV

    5.____

6. In a Christian funeral service, the pall is usually placed on the casket by

    6.____

A. the celebrant
B. an acolyte or acolytes
C. the crucifer
D. family members of the deceased

7. Which of the following is a cardiovascular manifestations associated with pulmonary edema?   7._____

   A. Slow, thready pulse
   B. Large Q waves
   C. Cyanosis
   D. Ejection click

8. Of the following sociological terms, _____ are considered similar to rituals and infused with symbolism.   8._____

   A. ceremonies
   B. folkways
   C. mores
   D. customs

9. A funeral service practitioner leases a funeral coach from a livery service. This type of bailment contract is referred to as   9._____

   A. adhesive
   B. iterative
   C. mutual benefit
   D. constructive

10. Most restorative work is performed after embalming, including   10._____
    I. removal of torn epidermis
    II. hypodermic tissue building of face and hands
    III. gluing disconnected tissues
    IV. hair restorations

    A. I and II
    B. II only
    C. II, III and IV
    D. I, II, III and IV

11. After a funeral service, in conversation with a funeral sendee practitioner, the mother of the deceased expresses the desire to receive grief counseling. The practitioner should recommend a   11._____

    A. group session
    B. psychologist
    C. preneed counselor
    D. hospital social worker

12. An embalming practitioner wants to make two gallons of 2% fluid. How many ounces of 32-index fluid will be needed?   12._____

A. 8
B. 16
C. 32
D. 64

13. An immunoglobulin is a

    A. carbohydrate
    B. glycoprotein
    C. protein
    D. nucleic acid

14. From the aorta toward the upper extremity, blood passes FIRST through the _____ artery.

    A. brachiocephalic
    B. subclavian
    C. axillary
    D. brachial

15. The Law of _____ is generally concerned with the scope of a buyer's authority.

    A. Agency
    B. Partnership
    C. Contract
    D. Torts

16. The best general stain remover for restoration purposes is

    A. acetone
    B. sodium hypochlorite
    C. benzene
    D. ether

17. Which of the following is likely to be influenced by the religious affiliation of the deceased?
    I. where the flowers are delivered
    II. where the funeral service is held
    III. which family member places the pall
    IV. the type of casket selected

    A. I and II
    B. I, II and III
    C. II and III
    D. I, II, III and IV

18. The primary difference between common law and statutory law, in terms of defining employee status, is that common law classifications

    A. are determined by industry best practices
    B. override statutory classifications
    C. are based on court decisions
    D. are specifically written into law

19. A recent widower states that he wants to move out of his house as soon as possible, to remove him and his children from the constant reminders of his late wife and their mother. The widower is failing to understand the experience common to most mourners, which is that

    A. moving is an experience that can only compound the stress of grief
    B. moving helps to sever important emotional bonds
    C. geography is not a factor that limits or controls memory
    D. absence makes the heart grow fonder

20. The main advantage of the direct selection room approach is that it

    A. enables the funeral director to better meet the needs of the family
    B. reduces the chance that the funeral director will misinterpret the body language of family members
    C. ensures the family's privacy during casket selection
    D. reduces the chance that the funeral director's presence will influence the family's choices

21. During the planning phase, a family member asks a funeral service practitioner about the benefit of viewing the deceased. The most appropriate reply to this inquiry would be that viewing

    A. is not usually recommended for people younger than 18 years of age
    B. may help others accept the reality of death
    C. is not likely to have much of an emotional impact
    D. is often a traumatic experience for those who were close to the deceased

22. The most desirable type of contract termination, from the contractor's point of view, is the

    A. default
    B. no-cost termination
    C. termination for convenience
    D. no-cost termination

23. Within a traditional Hopi native family, which typically exists as an extended patriarchal community, the person most likely to assume control of the family upon the father's death is the

    A. mother
    B. middle son
    C. eldest son
    D. mother's brother

24. Generally, a "non-guaranteed" preneed funeral contract specifies that the

    A. price of the funeral services and merchandise will not exceed the balance in the trust account at the time the funeral is provided
    B. arrangement may be canceled at any time, for any reason
    C. excess funds cannot be refunded if the amount in the trust account is less than the cost of the funeral
    D. funeral home will provide the funeral services and merchandise selected at the cost of those items at the time of the funeral

25. In most states, knowingly employing an unlicensed person in the practice of embalming is 25.____

　　A. against principles of professional practice, but legal
　　B. illegal
　　C. grounds for disciplinary action, only
　　D. an act leading to automatic suspension of licensure

KEY (CORRECT ANSWERS)

1.	C	11.	B
2.	A	12.	B
3.	D	13.	B
4.	A	14.	A
5.	C	15.	A
6.	D	16.	D
7.	C	17.	A
8.	A	18.	C
9.	C	19.	C
10.	C	20.	A

21. B
22. C
23. C
24. D
25. B

TEST 4

DIRECTIONS: Each question or incomplete statement is followed by several suggested answers or completions. Select the one that BEST answers the question or completes the statement. *PRINT THE LETTER OF THE CORRECT ANSWER IN THE SPACE AT THE RIGHT.*

1. Under FTC rules, the _____ Price List must be provided to each customer for their information and retention. 1._____

    A. Floral arrangement
    B. Casket
    C. Embalming
    D. General

2. The gross changes in proteins brought about by formaldehyde and other coagulating agents include 2._____
    I. decreased viscosity
    II. hardening
    III. resistance to digestion by enzymes
    IV. decreased water solubility

    A. I and II
    B. II only
    C. II, III and IV
    D. I, II, III and IV

3. In most areas of the country, no state or local law requires the purchase of a container to surround the casket in the grave. However, many cemeteries request the use of such a container so that 3._____

    A. the soil is not contaminated with leached embalming chemicals
    B. the grave cannot be easily dug up
    C. the grave will not sink in to the earth
    D. grave sites will be more clearly delineated

4. In Maslow's hierarchy of human needs, _____ needs must be met before all others. 4._____

    A. safety
    B. psychic
    C. biological
    D. self-esteem

5. In most jurisdictions, _____ CANNOT be included in the provisions of a preneed contract. 5._____
    I. markers
    II. sales funded by an insurance policy or an annuity contract
    III. interment rights in existing plots, crypts or niches
    IV. undelivered vaults

A. I only
B. I and IV
C. II and III
D. I, II, III and IV

6. Anticipatory grief is most likely to be associated with a person who dies of

    A. homicide
    B. SIDS
    C. cancer
    D. an automobile accident

7. Pathogenic microorganisms are usually most virulent

    A. in the presence of dry heat
    B. during the agonal period
    C. during the first 24 hours of an infection
    D. when they are first emitted from the body

8. In ancient Rome, the funeral sendee of a socially prominent person would most likely have been performed by one known as a

    A. libitinarius
    B. pontian
    C. vespillo
    D. curulis

9. In its pure state, formaldehyde is

    A. inert
    B. called "Formalin"
    C. a solid
    D. a gas

10. Some funeral directors use a _____ pricing system, which breaks charges down into several component parts such as professional service, facilities, automobile, and merchandise.

    A. itemized
    B. unit
    C. functional
    D. bi-unit

11. Early beliefs regarding death and the funeral rite, while diverse, suggest at least one common characteristic. Which of the following most accurately states this shared belief?

    A. The dead body is simply an empty shell that once contained a human soul.
    B. The body of the deceased should be attended with great care, often including a ritual washing.
    C. Death does not mark and end in the relationship between the living and the dead, but merely a transition in that relationship.
    D. The spiritual fate of the dead is, to varying degrees among cultures, dependent on the assiduousness of the survivors in performing the necessary rites.

12. Blood flowing to the arm and the hand travels FIRST through the _____ artery.

    A. radial
    B. axillary
    C. ulnar
    D. brachial

13. Of the following pairs of inflammatory cell types, _____ have almost identical functions and biochemical characteristics?

    A. Plasma cells and B lymphocytes
    B. Platelets and T lymphocytes
    C. Mast cells and basophils
    D. Monocytes and macrophages

14. In embalming, phenol solutions can be used for each of the following purposes, EXCEPT

    A. germicide
    B. hydrating
    C. bleaching
    D. preserving

15. A recently deceased person, admitted to a funeral home, is known to have had an infectious disease. The funeral director should inform
    I. the appropriate members of the funeral home staff
    II. public health officials
    III. close friends of the deceased
    IV. the appropriate law enforcement officials

    A. I only
    B. I and II
    C. II, III and IV
    D. I, II, III and IV

16. If excess skin is present around the margins of a wound, the most appropriate closure is the _____ suture.

    A. double intradermal
    B. baseball
    C. basket-weave
    D. worm

17. What is the term for a person or entity that undertakes to pay money or perform in the event that a principal fails to do so?

    A. Trustee
    B. Fiduciary
    C. Surety
    D. Guarantor

18. What is the term for the practice of adding a cost or expense to the basis of a property?

A. Averaging
B. Capitalization
C. Cost plus materials
D. Amortization

19. A people's basic patterns of thinking and acting, which are considered compulsory in nature, are known as

    A. mores
    B. folkways
    C. norms
    D. laws

20. OSHA regulations state that each occupational injury and illness must be recorded on Form 200 within _____ from the time the employer first learned of the injury or illness.

    A. 48 hours
    B. 6 working days
    C. 10 days
    D. 30 days

21. The body of research conducted by psychologists suggests that the human personality

    A. is a term used to refer to the deeper spiritual core of a person, rather than superficial aspects
    B. appears to be organized into patterns that are observable and measurable to some degree
    C. is solely a product of social and cultural environments, and has no biological or hereditary basis in biology
    D. involve s unique characteristics, none of which are shared with others

22. Most funeral service customers choose cremation because it is the alternative selected in advance by the deceased. The second most likely reason for selecting cremation is

    A. less emotional strain on the family
    B. the lower financial burden
    C. religious reasons
    D. environmental concerns

23. In the accounting cycle, the first entries are generally made in the

    A. journal
    B. ledger
    C. financial statements
    D. trial balance

24. The first step to Americans with Disabilities Act compliance is the

    A. site evaluation
    B. compliance statement
    C. priority list
    D. written compliance plan

25. A funeral service practitioner serves a family and provides both services and merchandise. The state requires the funeral home to pay 5% sales tax on merchandise. The charges for the family are as follows:
    Services $3000
    Casket $3250
    Vault $2000
    How much sales tax does the funeral director have to pay the state?

    A. $150
    B. $162.50
    C. $262.50
    D. $412.50

KEY (CORRECT ANSWERS)

1. D
2. C
3. C
4. C
5. C

6. C
7. D
8. A
9. D
10. C

11. C
12. B
13. C
14. B
15. A

16. D
17. C
18. B
19. A
20. B

21. B
22. B
23. A
24. A
25. C

TEST 5

DIRECTIONS: Each question or incomplete statement is followed by several suggested answers or completions. Select the one that BEST answers the question or completes the statement. *PRINT THE LETTER OF THE CORRECT ANSWER IN THE SPACE AT THE RIGHT.*

1. Under OSHA guidelines, the need for, and the type of, employee safety training is determined by the   1.____

   A. job description
   B. explicit personnel training policies of individual funeral homes
   C. generally accepted funeral home training practices
   D. employee's request for training

2. All aldehydes function by cross-linking   2.____

   A. fats
   B. salts
   C. hydrocarbons
   D. proteins

3. Each of the following is a facultative bacterium, EXCEPT   3.____

   A. coli
   B. Salmonella
   C. Staphylococcus aureus
   D. Listeria

4. As the body loses its ability to keep microorganisms in check during the agonal period, they move from one area to another in the body in a process known as   4.____

   A. necrosis
   B. algor mortis
   C. necrobiosis
   D. translocation

5. The majority of the microorganisms associated with the human body are   5.____

   A. bacteria
   B. viruses
   C. protozoa
   D. parasites

6. In accounting, the difference between the total debits and total credits is the   6.____

   A. trial balance
   B. balance
   C. revenue
   D. expense

7. Some groups, such as Tibetan Buddhist monks, or Zoroastrians, still follow the practice of exposing the dead to the elements, a method of disposal known as   7.____

A. sublimation
B. reincarnation
C. geomorphism
D. excarnation

8. Which of the following are MOST likely to experience an interstitial-to-plasma shift in fluids?

    A. Obese patients
    B. Post-surgical transplant patients
    C. Patients with a high fever
    D. Burn patients

9. In an acute bacterial infection, the neutrophil count in the blood is elevated, essentially because the neutrophils

    A. are following a chemotactic gradient
    B. have become activated
    C. are replicating in the blood
    D. are on their way from the bone marrow

10. The family of a deceased young woman gives to the funeral director a dress and jewelry to be placed on her body for the service. In legal terms, these items are considered _____ property.

    A. shared
    B. bailed
    C. loaned
    D. found

11. A computer's CPU contains the

    A. memory board
    B. mouse
    C. disk drive
    D. monitor

12. Long-term, uncontrolled diabetes mellitus often leads to

    A. Alzheimer's disease
    B. Guillain-Barre syndrome
    C. Hepatic neoplasms
    D. atherosclerosis

13. The exposure of embalming fluids to light results in
    I. opacity
    II. precipitation of endothermic solutes
    III. color changes
    IV. increased formaldehyde polymerization

    A. I only
    B. II and III
    C. III and IV
    D. I, II, III and IV

14. In the Eastern Orthodox Church, an image that is meant to represent a religious figure is known as a(n)   14.____

    A. hypostasis
    B. pantokrator
    C. icon
    D. theosis

15. Which of the following items can be listed on the General Price List as "free" or "no charge?"   15.____
    I. Casket seals
    II. Use of facilities for viewing
    III. Forwarding of remains to another funeral home
    IV. Transfer of remains to funeral home

    A. I only
    B. I and II
    C. III only
    D. None of these

16. The deceased has a cancerous growth on above his right eye. Which of the following restoration procedures would be performed LAST?   16.____

    A. Applying sealer to cavity walls
    B. Applying deep wound filler
    C. Applying surface restorer wax
    D. Drying subcutaneous surfaces

17. In posing the eyelids, the restorer should have them meet in   17.____

    A. the upper third of the eye socket
    B. the lower third of the eye socket
    C. the middle of the eye socket
    D. a line well below an imaginary line extending from the canthus

18. Each of the following is an appropriate source of temporary financing, EXCEPT   18.____

    A. term loans
    B. commercial paper
    C. accounts payable
    D. short-term notes

19. When arranging the floral displays next to the casket, it is generally accepted practice to place the   19.____

    A. largest arrangements nearest the casket
    B. arrangements that come in first nearest the casket
    C. family's flowers near the entrance
    D. family's flowers nearest the casket

20. Which of the following describes the most appropriate general lighting scheme for a casket display room?   20.____

A. Indirect, recessed incandescent light
B. Direct track lighting with incandescent bulbs
C. Recessed fluorescent bulbs with an opaque lens
D. Suspended fluorescent bulbs with a clear lens

21. For expensive caskets, the standard lining material is 21.____

    A. velvet
    B. satin
    C. silk
    D. linen

22. The Federal Trade Commission's Funeral Rule is an example of _____ law. 22.____

    A. statutory
    B. case
    C. common
    D. administrative

23. A seven-year-old girl has just lost her infant brother to SIDS. The funeral service practitioner, in working with the family, should advise the family 23.____

    A. to let the girl participate in the funeral
    B. that the girl probably does not have a clear understanding that death is final
    C. that the funeral will probably be a very traumatic experience for the girl
    D. to tell the child that her brother has gone to a better place

24. The ancient civilization whose funeral customs have been most influential on the practices and traditions of modern times was 24.____

    A. Mesopotamian
    B. Aztec
    C. Celtic
    D. Egyptian

25. In most states, the body of a person who dies an unattended death must 25.____

    A. be refrigerated for a certain period before disposition
    B. be buried as immediately as possible
    C. be identified by more than one family member
    D. undergo an autopsy

KEY (CORRECT ANSWERS)

1. A
2. D
3. A
4. D
5. A

6. B
7. D
8. D
9. D
10. B

11. A
12. D
13. C
14. C
15. D

16. C
17. B
18. C
19. D
20. A

21. A
22. D
23. A
24. D
25. D

EXAMINATION SECTION
TEST 1

DIRECTIONS: Each question or incomplete statement is followed by several suggested answers or completions. Select the one that BEST answers the question or completes the statement. *PRINT THE LETTER OF THE CORRECT ANSWER IN THE SPACE AT THE RIGHT.*

1. The United States, each of the following is an overall demographic trend regarding mortality, EXCEPT

    A. in every group up to age eighty, nonwhite mortality is higher than white mortality
    B. men live approximately seven years longer than women
    C. the death rates of a given demographic tend to go down as that group's occupational prestige rises
    D. married people have lower mortality rates than single people

    1.____

2. When leading family members into the viewing room for their first viewing of the deceased, which of the following approaches would be recommended?

    A. Lead the family slowly to the casket and then stand next to the deceased and ask whether any changes in appearance need to be made.
    B. Stay away from the viewing room entirely, and let the family know they may enter when they are comfortable doing so.
    C. Escort the family about halfway into the room, and then stand back as they approach the casket.
    D. Lead the family slowly to the casket, indicate that they may come forward for the viewing, and then immediately leave the room.

    2.____

3. What is the Hebrew term for the ritual washing of the deceased's body before burial?

    A. Midrash
    B. Taharah
    C. Kippot
    D. Sheva

    3.____

4. What type of chemical is used to increase the capability of embalmed tissues to retain moisture?

    A. Humectant
    B. Preservative
    C. Surfactant
    D. Osmotic

    4.____

5. Each of the following is a physical technique that the embalming practitioner can use to improve the distribution of arterial solution, EXCEPT

    A. massaging along arterial routes
    B. a single sustained, steady injection of constant flow
    C. restricting drainage
    D. increasing the pressure of the arterial solution

    5.____

6. In order for an offer to be valid under contract law, it must
   I. be clearly communicated to the offeree
   II. be complete and clear
   III. seriously express the intent to contract
   IV. be in writing

   A. I only   B. I, II and III   C. II and IIV   D. I, II, III and IV

7. Which of the following is a term for the abnormal fear of death or corpses?

   A. Camophobia   B. Thanatophilia   C. Adduction   D. Necrophobia

8. A liturgical church is shaped like a(n)

   A. tricorn   B. oval   C. circle   D. cross

9. Which of the following is NOT typically a pre-embalming restorative procedure?

   A. Mouth and lip closure
   B. Shaving of facial hair
   C. Alignment of lacerated tissue edges
   D. Firming and setting facial tissues

10. A(n) _____ preneed contract is necessary if an applicant wants to qualify for Social Security and Medicaid funeral benefits.

    A. compounding   B. irrevocable   C. revocable   D. guaranteed

11. Which of the following is an on-line application that locates and displays the document associated with a hyperlink?

    A. plug-in   B. finder   C. server   D. browser

12. Each of the following is a reason why hardwood caskets often cost more than metal caskets, EXCEPT

    A. species availability   B. expected durability
    C. the amount of workmanship   D. variable costs

13. An emaciated appearance at the temple can be corrected with the injection of filler from one of several hidden injection points. Which of the following is NOT one of these injection points?

    A. The eyebrow   B. The hair of the temple
    C. Behind the anterior helix   D. Below the orbital bone

14. The cecum is located in the _____ region.

    A. right inguinal   B. left inguinal
    C. right lumbar   D. left lumbar

15. What is the term for the stand on which the casket rests while in state and during the funeral service?   15.____

   A. Precipice   B. Altar   C. Mortar   D. Catafalque

16. Spouses employed by the same employer   16.____

   A. may be limited to twelve weeks annual leave in the aggregate for the birth or adoption of a child or to care for a sick parent
   B. must take their leave at the same time
   C. may not take leave at the same time
   D. are each granted twelve weeks annual leave in the aggregate for the birth or adoption of a child or to care for a sick parent

17. The thickness of copper and bronze caskets is most commonly expressed in terms of   17.____

   A. standard gauge
   B. fractions of an inch
   C. ounces per square foot
   D. number of sheets per inch

18. What is the legal term for false statements that are made in writing for the purpose of injuring the reputation of another?   18.____

   A. Libel   B. Aspersion   C. Slander   D. Calumny

19. A funeral service practitioner signs a contract requiring merchandise to be delivered to his funeral home without his incurring any expense for the delivery. This agreement is described as   19.____

   A. cost and freight   B. COD
   C. last in, first out   D. advance charges

20. The FTC's funeral rule requires or allows that   20.____

   A. an Outer Burial Container Price List may be omitted from the General Price List
   B. the prices on a General Price List must be itemized
   C. prices be discussed initially in the casket room
   D. the funeral home may charge for embalming in any case it desires

21. During preneed counseling, a 70-year-old woman who has lived alone for the past twelve years tells the funeral service practitioner that her life has been a series of unmet goals. According to the model of psychosocial development proposed by Erik Erikson, the woman illustrates the stage of   21.____

   A. intimacy vs. isolation
   B. integrity vs. despair
   C. generativity vs. stagnation
   D. basic trust vs. mistrust

22. The Federal Trade Commission specifically requires the provision of each of the following, EXCEPT the

    A. Funeral Agreement Form
    B. Casket Rice List
    C. Statement of Funeral Goods and Services Selected
    D. Outer Burial Container Price List

23. In the _____ price structure, there is an inverse relationship between the markup and the price of a casket.

    A. fixed multiple
    B. graduated recovery
    C. quartiled
    D. declining price

24. Which of the following viruses is always detectable after infections?

    A. Hepatitis B
    B. Cytomegalovirus
    C. Varicella-zoster
    D. Herpes simplex

25. The "24 hour law" in most states requires that one of four things must be done with a body within 24 hours of death. Which of the following is NOT one of these?

    A. Burial
    B. Cremation
    C. Refrigeration, typically below 40 degrees F
    D. Embalming

KEY (CORRECT ANSWERS)

1.	B	11.	D
2.	C	12.	B
3.	B	13.	D
4.	A	14.	A
5.	B	15.	D
6.	B	16.	A
7.	D	17.	C
8.	D	18.	A
9.	D	19.	D
10.	B	20.	C

21. B
22. A
23. A
24. A
25. B

TEST 2

DIRECTIONS: Each question or incomplete statement is followed by several suggested answers or completions. Select the one that BEST answers the question or completes the statement. *PRINT THE LETTER OF THE CORRECT ANSWER IN THE SPACE AT THE RIGHT.*

1. A casket that is fully opened at the head and foot is described as

    A. uncapped
    B. full couch
    C. single hinged
    D. single panel

2. Of the fungi that cause disease in compromised hosts, the most widely distributed are

    A. Candida
    B. Pneumocystis
    C. Aspergillus
    D. Blastomyces

3. In 1994, the Federal Trade Commission amended the Funeral Rule and added the provision that funeral directors were required to

    A. provide price lists for caskets and other products
    B. inform customers that embalming is a legal requirement
    C. standardize the definition of a "protective" casket
    D. accept caskets that families procure on their own

4. Which of the following is NOT a major type of preservative used in embalming fluids?

    A. Phenols
    B. Esters
    C. Aldehydes
    D. Alcohols

5. If a family wants a sealed outer burial container to protect the casket, the best option would be a

    A. triune
    B. grave liner
    C. Ziegler case
    D. vault

6. The medical term for a black eye is

    A. ptosis
    B. ecchymosis
    C. edema
    D. periorbit

7. The merchandise and supplies on hand at any given time in a funeral home are listed in the record known as the

   A. inventory
   B. ledger
   C. balance sheet
   D. journal

   7.____

8. In the embalming of the normal adult body, the order of injection sites typically begins with the

   A. right and left subclavian arteries
   B. right and left common carotid arteries
   C. right femoral artery
   D. aortic arch

   8.____

9. A person who dies without having made a valid will is said to have died

   A. intestate
   B. insolvent
   C. in probate
   D. holographically

   9.____

10. A computer operating system's overall quality is most often judged on its ability to manage

    A. peripheral drivers
    B. disk utilities
    C. file backup
    D. program execution

    10.____

11. The Hebrew term for the period of mourning that lasts for a year after one's death is

    A. shemirah
    B. tallith
    C. aveilut
    D. tachrichim

    11.____

12. Which of the following is a humectant?

    A. Citric acid
    B. Sorbitol
    C. Sodium lauryl sulfate
    D. Methanol

    12.____

13. According to Watson and Tellegen's "map" of the structure of human emotions, the emotions that are most closely related are

    A. anger and fear
    B. love and hate
    C. disappointment and relief
    D. pleasure and pain

    13.____

14. A handshake is an example of a

    A. ceremony
    B. norm
    C. more
    D. folkway

15. HIV infection will result in a depletion of _____ cells.

    A. $CD1^+$
    B. $CD2^+$
    C. $CD3^+$
    D. $CD4+$

16. For what reason is chromium frequently added to carbon steel?

    A. To reduce rust and corrosion
    B. To reduce cost
    C. To impart a higher gloss
    D. To add strength

17. Which of the following species of wood might be used to make a softwood casket?

    A. Maple
    B. Oak
    C. Pine
    D. Cherry

18. Third-space (edemic) fluid is called "exudate" if it contains

    A. protein
    B. glucose
    C. water
    D. red blood cells

19. The system of venous injection that was a precursor of modern embalming procedures was developed by

    A. Galen
    B. Confucius
    C. Hippocrates
    D. Leonardo Da Vinci

20. _____ is the process by which the social values of the funeral rite are most commonly learned.

    A. Enculturation
    B. Religion
    C. Assimilation
    D. Indoctrination

21. What is the term for the purplish-red discoloration of the skin that is caused by the accumulation of blood in the lower portions of a deceased's body?   21.____

    A. Necrolividity
    B. Cyanosis
    C. Livor mortis
    D. Rigor mortis

22. A funeral service practitioner is LEAST likely to use a hearse in the transfer of or removal of the deceased's remains when the deceased   22.____

    A. is elderly
    B. has died of a communicable disease
    C. is an infant
    D. died in a hospital or nursing home

23. A contractual agreement to have the subject of a sale delivered to a designated place, usually either the place of shipment or the place of destination, without expense to the buyer, is described as   23.____

    A. a specific performance
    B. free on board
    C. quantum meruit
    D. a contract of bailment

24. Which of the following is a benign neoplasm found in the blood?   24.____

    A. Lymphangioma
    B. Leiomyoma
    C. Hemangioma
    D. Glioma

25. To smooth wax or clean the hair, a restorative artist would typically use   25.____

    A. phenol
    B. tissue builder solvent
    C. undiluted cavity fluid
    D. acetone

KEY (CORRECT ANSWERS)

1. B	11. C
2. C	12. B
3. D	13. A
4. B	14. D
5. D	15. D
6. C	16. A
7. A	17. C
8. B	18. A
9. A	19. D
10. D	20. A

21. C
22. C
23. B
24. C
25. D

TEST 3

DIRECTIONS: Each question or incomplete statement is followed by several suggested answers or completions. Select the one that BEST answers the question or completes the statement PRINT THE LETTER OF THE CORRECT ANSWER IN THE SPACE AT THE RIGHT.

1. Which of the following would be useful for reducing swelling in a localized area? 1.____

    A. Electric spatula
    B. Undercoat
    C. Mastic compress
    D. Armature

2. The style of casket interior in which the material is drawn or gathered in parallel fashion is 2.____

    A. tufted   B. shirred   C. carriage   D. crushed

3. The average shelf life of embalming fluids is typically 3.____

    A. 9 to 18 months
    B. 1 to 3 years
    C. 2 to 5 years
    D. 10 to 15 years

4. A person having a legal duty to act primarily for the benefit of another is a(n) 4.____

    A. fiduciary   B. guardian   C. obligor   D. ward

5. A typical funeral home cortege is led by the 5.____

    A. hearse
    B. closest family member's car
    C. pallbearer's car
    D. funeral home car, with clergy

6. A business partnership generally 6.____

    A. is led by a senior partner has total control of decision-making
    B. does not pay income tax
    C. generally has the same limited liability of a corporation
    D. can consist of many shareholders

7. The computer's hardware/software interface is the 7.____

    A. buffer
    B. bus
    C. application
    D. operating system

8. In the galvanizing process, steel is coated with 8.____

    A. zinc   B. lead   C. aluminum   D. tin

9. Which of the following is a superficial fungal infection of the skin that tends to intensify when associated with AIDS? 9.____

    A. Histoplasmosis
    B. Candidiasis
    C. Tinea corporis
    D. Ringworm

63

10. A funeral service practitioner discovers that a family members was intoxicated when she signed the contractual portion of the funeral agreement. The contract is therefore

    A. unenforceable
    B. voidable
    C. void
    D. valid

11. It is most appropriate for the funeral service practitioner to explain and discuss the medical terminology used on a person's death certificate

    A. during preneed arrangements
    B. when the family members ask
    C. upon the first meeting with the family
    D. at the committal service

12. What is the total interest received on a 10%, 90-day note for $ 1500?

    A. $37.50   B. $50   C. $75   D. $87.50

13. According to Jean Piaget, a person's understanding of the need for social norms is clearest if they are learned from the

    A. political leaders or government authorities
    B. religioas authorities
    C. parents
    D. peer group

14. A contract must be _____ in order to be enforced by courts.

    A. valid   B. written   C. voidable   D. bonded

15. During embalming, the presence of a thrombus would be evidenced by

    A. desquamation
    B. edema
    C. diminished distribution
    D. staining

16. Of the following, which is an example of a signed agreement of an oral understanding?

    A. Embalming authorization
    B. Floral arrangements
    C. Request for military honors
    D. Music selections

17. In a civil action, _____ amages are those paid over and above the actual loss.

    A. punitive
    B. liquidated
    C. compensatory
    D. moratory

18. Among the main chemicals common to almost all embalming preservative solutions are formaldehyde and   18._____

    A. ammonium compounds
    B. ethyl alcohol
    C. water
    D. nitrates

19. The metal liner sometimes used to prevent leakage inside a vessel that contains a body, especially during shipping, is known as a   19._____

    A. transfer container
    B. Ziegler case
    C. scupper
    D. triune

20. The casket of a layperson, in a Roman Catholic funeral Mass, is usually placed   20._____

    A. with the feet toward the choir rail
    B. parallel to the altar
    C. with the head toward the altar
    D. with the feet toward the altar

21. Families, like individuals, frequently respond to stress by   21._____

    A. decompensating to the lowest level of individual functioning
    B. projecting a false self
    C. mobilizing resources and promoting each member's welfare
    D. becoming stuck in rigid, dysfunctional patterns

22. The _____ family is likely to be most acutely affected by the death of a child.   22._____

    A. extended
    B. intergenerational
    C. joint
    D. nuclear

23. Anisocytosis is a term that refers to variation in the _____ of red blood cells.   23._____

    A. function
    B. size
    C. synthesis
    D. shape

24. Which of the following is NOT an *artery* that is used in the six-point injection process?   24._____

    A. Left common carotid
    B. Right axial
    C. Right subclavian
    D. Left femoral

25. The "minimal services" provision of the FTC Funeral Rule require that funeral service providers list a minimum of four service items on their General Price List. Which of the following is NOT one of these four "minimal sendees?"

    A. Use of facilities and staff for viewing
    B. Direct cremation
    C. Forwarding of remains
    D. Immediate burial

KEY (CORRECT ANSWERS)

1. A
2. B
3. C
4. A
5. D

6. B
7. D
8. A
9. B
10. B

11. B
12. A
13. D
14. A
15. C

16. A
17. A
18. B
19. B
20. D

21. D
22. D
23. B
24. C
25. A

TEST 4

DIRECTIONS: Each question or incomplete statement is followed by several suggested answers or completions. Select the one that BEST answers the question or completes the statement. *PRINT THE LETTER OF THE CORRECT ANSWER IN THE SPACE AT THE RIGHT.*

1. The first stage of anticipatory grief, described by Kübler-Ross, is 1.____

   A. bargaining
   B. anger
   C. depression
   D. denial

2. Which of the following is typically incorporated into embalming fluid as an antipolymerization agent? 2.____

   A. Methanol
   B. Water
   C. Glycerin
   D. Sodium citrate

3. Which of the following is NOT a lining material used in caskets? 3.____

   A. Masselin
   B. Linen
   C. Velvet
   D. Crepe

4. What is the term for a business or individual to whom a debt is owed? 4.____

   A. Creditor
   B. Debtor
   C. Lien holder
   D. Drawee

5. Which of the following is secondarily liable on a promissory note? 5.____

   A. Endorser
   B. Maker
   C. Endorsee
   D. Payee

6. The _____ host is the host on which a parasitic organism either attains sexual maturity or reproduces. 6.____

   A. final
   B. transfer
   C. secondary
   D. replicative

7. Legally, inventory is classified as

    A. real property
    B. an intangible asset
    C. tangible personal property
    D. intangible personal property

8. A human attribute that is deeply discrediting, and thus makes a person less desirable from others, is known as a(n)

    A. stigma
    B. idiosyncrasy
    C. taboo
    D. stereotype

9. Adding the beginning merchandise inventory to the purchases for the period yields the

    A. cost of merchandise sold
    B. gross purchases
    C. cost of goods available for sale
    D. net sales

10. Casket bearers, when placing a casket on a grave-lowering device, should grasp the handle by the

    A. arm
    B. bar
    C. point
    D. lug

11. Of the following, the first to decompose following death is the

    A. sclera
    B. tracheal lining
    C. mesentery
    D. colon

12. What is the term for a burial container that is broader at the shoulders than at the head or feet?

    A. Casket
    B. Drage
    C. Coffin
    D. Catafalque

13. A funeral service practitioner is generally liable for accidents that occur in each of the following locations, EXCEPT the

    A. religious facility where the funeral service is held
    B. site where the death has occurred
    C. cemetery
    D. funeral home, during visitation or services

14. The family of a recently deceased young man asks the funeral director whether she thinks they should order an autopsy. The funeral director should

    A. advise them to consult their physician
    B. explain in detail what is involved in an autopsy
    C. tell them an autopsy is rarely required by law
    D. encourage the autopsy if the death seems suspicious

15. In the embalming process, the method most commonly used to open the artery or vein is to make a _____ incision into the vessel.

    A. diagonal
    B. transverse
    C. T-shaped
    D. wedge

16. What is the term for personal property that is permanently attached to land?

    A. Buildings
    B. Real estate
    C. Deed
    D. Fixture

17. In application software, utilities such as the spelling checker are typically included in the _____ menu.

    A. help
    B. macros
    C. file
    D. tools

18. The "peak experience" described in Abraham Maslow's Hierarchy of Needs is

    A. status
    B. safety
    C. self-actualization
    D. love and belonging

19. Among all types of infectious renal disorders, the most common causative organism is

    A. E. coli
    B. Salmonella
    C. Pseudomonas
    D. Staphylococcus

20. "Client-centered" counseling is essentially

    A. solution-focused
    B. nondirective
    C. crisis-oriented
    D. psychoanalytical

21. To address _____ in the body of the deceased, the embalming practitioner often uses the post-embalming technique of hypodermic tissue building.

    A. livor mortis
    B. gas buildup
    C. edema
    D. emaciation

22. Post-traumatic stress disorder is classified as a(n) _____ disorder.

    A. personality
    B. anxiety
    C. dissociative
    D. mood

23. Which of the following is a legal term describing a contract in which a dominant party has taken unfair advantage of a weaker party?

    A. Voidable
    B. Unilateral
    C. Adhesive
    D. Unconscionable

24. The deceased has a cancerous growth on her lower left cheek. Which of the following restoration procedures would be performed FIRST?

    A. Injecting surrounding tissues with preservative or cavity fluid
    B. Embalming the body
    C. Applying surface restorer wax
    D. Excising the tumor

25. If a funeral home has not served a family before, the most likely reason a person will choose that particular home's services is the home's

    A. recommendation by a third party
    B. proximity to their residence
    C. religious affiliation
    D. reputation

KEY (CORRECT ANSWERS)

1. D
2. A
3. A
4. A
5. A

6. A
7. C
8. A
9. C
10. B

11. B
12. C
13. B
14. A
15. B

16. D
17. D
18. C
19. A
20. B

21. D
22. B
23. D
24. B
25. B

TEST 5

DIRECTIONS: Each question or incomplete statement is followed by several suggested answers or completions. Select the one that BEST answers the question or completes the statement. *PRINT THE LETTER OF THE CORRECT ANSWER IN THE SPACE AT THE RIGHT.*

1. On a casket, a _____ handle is a single handle in which the lug, arm, and bar are combined in one unit.

    A. convertible
    B. welded
    C. swing
    D. bail

2. Most sociologists consider the root of all cultural systems to be

    A. economics
    B. religion
    C. language
    D. family

3. Most state laws require that a certain period—usually 48 hours—must follow a person's death before his or her body can be

    A. embalmed
    B. refrigerated
    C. cremated
    D. buried

4. Each of the following is a buffer commonly used in embalming fluid, EXCEPT

    A. methanol
    B. sodium citrate
    C. borax
    D. sodium phosphate

5. The person who files a lawsuit in court is known as the

    A. plaintiff
    B. legatee
    C. class actor
    D. defendant

6. The only service fee that the Federal Trade Commission allows to be nondeclinable at the outset of a funeral transaction is the fee for

    A. basic services for funeral director and staff
    B. the use of vehicles
    C. embalming
    D. the use of facilities

7. According to Wolfelt, the funeral service practitioner establishes a helping relationship with a family using the following steps. The proper sequence of these steps is:
   I. Building a relationship with the family
   II. Implementing the funeral arrangements
   III. Consolidating and planning the funeral arrangements
   IV. Helping the family understand alternatives

   A. I, III, IV, II
   B. IV, I, III, II
   C. I, IV, III, II
   D. I, II, IV, III

8. _____ is defined as the evacuation of gases, liquids, and semisolids from a natural body orifice.

   A. Purge
   B. Leakage
   C. Desquamation
   D. Flatus

9. In the manufacture of caskets, kapok is used as a _____ material.

   A. padding
   B. backing
   C. lining
   D. casket covering

10. In a funeral cortege, drivers under the direction of the funeral director are legally referred to as _____ drivers.

    A. contract
    B. insider
    C. agent
    D. livery

11. The practice of embalming was not widely used by U.S. morticians until

    A. the War of 1812
    B. the Civil War
    C. the Spanish-American War
    D. World War I

12. For long, dense, and more extensive hair restorations, _____ affords the strongest bond.

    A. suturing
    B. wax
    C. embedding
    D. cement

13. A(n) _____ contract is typically used when uncertainties in contract performance do not permit costs to be estimated with sufficient accuracy.   13.____

    A. requirements
    B. cost-reimbursement
    C. time-and-materials
    D. indefinite-quantity

14. The standard government headstone used on the gravesites of many buried military veterans is ultimately the property of the   14.____

    A. family of the deceased
    B. U.S. government
    C. state government
    D. cemetery where the veteran is buried

15. In considering the mode of action of an antimicrobial compound, an important factor should be   15.____

    A. plasmid-mediated resistance
    B. transposition
    C. selective toxicity
    D. cross-resistance

16. _____ is the proper term used to describe the placing of cremated remains in a final container.   16.____

    A. sepulture
    B. inurnment
    C. interment
    D. funeration

17. To close an abdominal puncture wound, an embalming practitioner typically uses a type of suture known as the _____ stitch.   17.____

    A. baseball
    B. single intradermal
    C. worm
    D. purse string

18. A(n) _____ funeral rite is one that is adjusted to the needs and wants of those who are directly involved in the service.   18.____

    A. humanistic
    B. secular
    C. adaptive
    D. non-denominational

19. A culture's mandatory prescriptions against certain acts are referred to as   19.____

    A. mores
    B. laws
    C. norms
    D. taboos

20. What is the medical term for inflammation of the sac surrounding the heart?

    A. Myocarditis
    B. Endocarditis
    C. Fibrillation
    D. Pericarditis

21. Which of the following terms is used to describe the degree to which people are comfortable with ambiguous situations and with the inability to accurately predict future events?

    A. uncertainty avoidance
    B. mental set
    C. cognitive dissonance
    D. thematic apperception

22. Each of the following functions can be performed with a spreadsheet application, EXCEPT

    A. fiscal forecasting
    B. budget charts and graphs
    C. audiovisual presentations
    D. inventory management

23. Each of the following is a feature of a limited liability partnership, EXCEPT that

    A. limited partners may not participate in the management of the company
    B. all partners have limited liability
    C. it is taxed the same as a regular partnership
    D. the names of limited partners may not appear in the company's name

24. Which of the following is NOT typically used as a deep filler during restoration?

    A. Mastic
    B. Sealer-impregnated cotton
    C. Soft wax
    D. Piaster of Paris

25. In the Hindu tradition, after death the body of the deceased is placed on the ground with the head pointing

    A. east
    B. west
    C. south
    D. north

KEY (CORRECT ANSWERS)

1. D
2. C
3. C
4. A
5. A

6. A
7. C
8. A
9. A
10. C

11. B
12. D
13. B
14. B
15. C

16. B
17. D
18. C
19. D
20. D

21. A
22. C
23. B
24. C
25. C

EXAMINATION SECTION

TEST 1

DIRECTIONS: Each question or incomplete statement is followed by several suggested answers or completions. Select the one that BEST answers the question or completes the statement. *PRINT THE LETTER OF THE CORRECT ANSWER IN THE SPACE AT THE RIGHT.*

1. Which of the following is NOT required to be on the General Price List?
    A. Casket price list
    B. Embalming charges
    C. Use of automotive equipment
    D. Transportation of remains to the funeral home

2. According to the OSHA, the medical record for each employee shall be preserved and maintained for at least the duration of employment plus _____ years.
    A. 10   B. 20   C. 30   D. 40

3. Which of the following are similar to rituals and charged with symbolic content?
    A. Customs
    B. Folkways
    C. Ceremonies
    D. Initiations

4. Clothes and jewelry given to the funeral director to be placed on the dead body are considered in law as
    A. no property
    B. quasi-property
    C. bailed property
    D. unclaimed property

5. Which of the following regarding the Federal Trade Commission (FTC) requirements is true?
    A. Prices are initially discussed in the casket display room
    B. An Outer Burial Container Price List is not a requirement
    C. A General Price List must have all prices itemized
    D. A funeral home may require embalming on all cases

6. When consulted by the family concerning the advisability of an autopsy, the funeral director should
    A. encourage it
    B. discourage it
    C. explain in detail what it involves
    D. advise they confer with their physician

7. To qualify for Supplemental Security Income (SSI) and Medicaid benefits, applicants purchasing preneed funerals must enter into which of the following preneed contracts?
    A. Revocable
    B. Guaranteed
    C. Irrevocable
    D. Nonguaranteed

7._____

8. When explaining casket differences to a family, the term *protective* indicates that the casket
    A. preserves the body from decomposition
    B. is constructed of an impermeable material
    C. will not require an outer burial container
    D. is designed to resist the entrance of outside elements

8._____

9. What is the interest on a $1,000 note for 3 months at a 9% annual interest rate?
    A. $15.00
    B. $18.50
    C. $22.50
    D. $30.00

9._____

10. If the deceased had an infectious disease, the funeral director should only inform the appropriate
    A. friends
    B. members of the staff
    C. members of the clergy
    D. members of law enforcement agencies

10._____

11. Embalming came into wide practice in the United States during
    A. the Revolutionary War
    B. the War of 1812
    C. the Civil War
    D. World War I

11._____

12. Under the American with Disabilities Act (ADA), when a death is due to AIDS (HIV), the funeral home may
    I. require a sealed casket
    II. have a public viewing
    III. charge more for embalming
    IV. have a private service

    A. I and II only
    B. I and III only
    C. II and IV only
    D. III and IV only

12._____

13. If the thickness of ferrous caskets is reported as gauge, a casket 1/16-inch thick would be _____ gauge. 13._____
    A. 8 B. 16 C. 32 D. 48

14. A humanistic service would be a(n) 14._____
    A. service at a mosque
    B. Masonic Lodge service
    C. Elks Lodge service with prayers
    D. service with no religious connotation

15. Placement of the pall on the casket should be done at the direction of the 15._____
    A. acolyte
    B. crucifer
    C. clergyperson
    D. family of the deceased

16. Which of the following religious groups prohibit cremation? 16._____
    A. Buddhists and Hindus
    B. Orthodox Jews and Muslims
    C. Roman Catholics and Sikhs
    D. Reform Jews and Christians

17. In comparing a 16- and 20-gauge steel casket, the 16-gauge casket would be 17._____
    A. thicker and heavier
    B. thinner and lighter
    C. thicker but less durable
    D. thicker with no weight difference

18. What price list must be offered to each customer for their information and retention? 18._____
    A. Casket B. Flower
    C. General D. Cash Advance

19. A Greek Orthodox religious picture is called a(n) 19._____
    A. kever B. icon C. solea D. trisagion

20. When explaining casket shell designs to a family, which of the following is an end or corner design? 20._____
    A. Shirred B. Elliptic
    C. Crinkled D. Galvanized

21. A dead body is in one mortuary. A second mortuary that has control of the final disposition is said to have
    A. actual custody
    B. present custody
    C. contract of possession
    D. constructive possession

22. The proper terminology for the placing of cremated remains into a final container is
    A. interment
    B. inurnment
    C. entombment
    D. cremains interment

23. A practitioner enters into a helping relationship with a family. According to Wolfelt, what is the order of the phases for the practitioner to use in establishing this relationship?
    I. Assist the family in understanding their alternatives
    II. Consolidate and plan the funeral arrangements
    III. Build the relationship with the family
    IV. Implement the funeral arrangements

    A. II, III, IV, I
    B. III, I, II, IV
    C. III, II, I, IV
    D. IV, I, II, III

24. Which of the following is the shape of a liturgical church?
    A. oval   B. cross   C. square   D. octagon

25. Personal property permanently attached to land is known as
    A. quitclaim   B. premium
    C. novation   D. fixture

KEY (CORRECT ANSWERS)

1. C	11. C	21. C
2. A	12. B	22. B
3. A	13. B	23. B
4. C	14. B	24. B
5. C	15. C	25. D
6. D	16. B	
7. C	17. A	
8. D	18. C	
9. C	19. B	
10. B	20. B	

TEST 2

DIRECTIONS: Each question or incomplete statement is followed by several suggested answers or completions. Select the one that BEST answers the question or completes the statement. *PRINT THE LETTER OF THE CORRECT ANSWER IN THE SPACE AT THE RIGHT.*

1. A debit to the purchases account would have a corresponding credit in which of the following accounts?
    A. Inventory
    B. Sales expense
    C. Accounts payable
    D. Accounts receivable

    1._____

2. If the total of expenses is smaller than the total of revenues, the difference is termed
    A. net worth
    B. net profit
    C. gross profit
    D. gross margin

    2._____

3. Survivors of a traumatic event involving the sudden death of others should
    A. rely on medications
    B. avoid joining a support group
    C. think about it, but not discuss it
    D. talk about the event when the subject arises

    3._____

4. Which of the following has occurred if a funeral service practitioner intentionally misrepresents a benefit of a preneed funeral arrangement?
    A. Fraud   B. Duress
    C. Mistake   D. Under influence

    4._____

5. A preneed contract that may be terminated by the purchaser at any time before the death of the beneficiary, with a refund of the monies paid as prescribed by state law, is
    A. revocable   B. guaranteed
    C. irrevocable   D. nonguaranteed

    5._____

6. Which of the following is the correct sequence of accounting procedures?
    A. ledger, trial balance, journal, financial statements
    B. journal, ledger, trial balance, financial statements
    C. financial statements, trial balance, ledger, journal
    D. financial statements, journal, ledger, trial balance

    6._____

7. The religious affiliation of a deceased may play a role in
   I. type of casket selected
   II. location of the funeral service
   III. where the flowers are delivered
   IV. which family member places the pall on the casket

   A. I and II only
   B. I and IV only
   C. II and III only
   D. III and IV only

8. In order to transport casketed remains 3,000 miles away, the practitioner should
   A. get permission from the church elders
   B. contact the Social Security Administration
   C. make arrangements with a common carrier
   D. place a paid obituary notice in the local newspaper

9. When is it appropriate to explain and discuss medical terminology used on the death certificate?
   A. When making the removal
   B. At the committal service
   C. When the family inquires
   D. During preneed arrangements

10. The person who brings an action in court is the
    A. plaintiff
    B. litigatee
    C. defendant
    D. legatee

11. Requirements for a valid offer must
    I. include a specific time duration
    II. include an acceptance
    III. be definite
    IV. be seriously intended

    A. I, II and III only
    B. I, II and IV only
    C. I, III and IV only
    D. II, III and IV only

12. A business or individual to whom a debt is owed is a
    A. drawee   B. drawer   C. debtor   D. creditor

13. A typical 6-year-old child whose parents have died may
    I. accept that death is final and inevitable
    II. have no comprehension of death
    III. fail to adequately mourn
    IV. try to personify death

    A. I and II only
    B. I and IV only
    C. II and III only
    D. III and IV only

14. According to Bowlby, the four aspects of the attachment theory are
    A. involvement, despair, reliance and strength of attachment
    B. powerfulness of attachment, reliance, despair and threat of loss
    C. strength of attachment, security of attachment, reliance and involvement
    D. despair, threat of loss, security of attachment and strength of attachment

15. In order for a contract to be enforced by the courts, it must be
    A. void
    B. valid
    C. voidable
    D. unenforceable

16. Funeral claims against the decedent's estate are
    A. secondary claims
    B. preferred claims
    C. illegal when filed
    D. treated as any other debt

17. The feeling that one's own cultural responses and activities relative to death are superior to those of other cultures is an example of
    A. ethnocentrism
    B. cultural universal
    C. cultural relativism
    D. an adaptive funeral rite

18. The Roman undertaker was called the
    A. Praeco
    B. Naidia
    C. Kherheb
    D. Libitinarius

19. The difference between the total debits and total credits in an account is the
    A. balance
    B. expense
    C. revenue
    D. trial balance

20. Galvanizing is a process in which steel is coated with
    A. tin   B. iron   C. zinc   D. copper

21. A family member asks about the benefit of viewing the deceased. The best reply would be that viewing
    A. is required by law
    B. has no emotional impact
    C. helps with the acceptance of reality
    D. is necessary for identification

22. The most commonly accepted means of measuring thickness of copper and bronze caskets is
    A. ounces per square inch
    B. ounces per square foot
    C. number of sheets per inch
    D. number of sheets per foot

23. The state or condition of dying without having made a valid will is called
    A. testate   B. intestate
    C. insolvency   D. holographic will

24. Ultimately, the standard government headstone or marker is the property of the
    A. family
    B. cemetery
    C. Social Security Administration
    D. Veterans Affairs

25. Adding the beginning merchandise inventory to the purchases for the period yields
    A. gross sales
    B. net purchases
    C. cost of merchandise sold
    D. goods available for sales

KEY (CORRECT ANSWERS)

1. C	11. C	21. C
2. B	12. D	22. B
3. D	13. C	23. B
4. A	14. C	24. B
5. A	15. B	25. D
6. B	16. D	
7. B	17. A	
8. C	18. D	
9. C	19. A	
10. A	20. C	

TEST 3

DIRECTIONS: Each question or incomplete statement is followed by several suggested answers or completions. Select the one that BEST answers the question or completes the statement. *PRINT THE LETTER OF THE CORRECT ANSWER IN THE SPACE AT THE RIGHT.*

1. In a well-managed funeral home, the source of acceptable employee procedures is the
    A. employer's mandate
    B. employee's coworkers
    C. employee's own judgment
    D. up-to-date employee handbook

    1._____

2. Which of the following are correct about the value of a funeral rite to a family?
    I. provides an emotional outlet
    II. provides a way to avoid the grieving process
    III. provides psychological benefits
    IV. causes a division in the family

    A. I and III only
    B. I and IV only
    C. II and III only
    D. II and IV only

    2._____

3. An irrevocable funded preneed funeral contract stipulates that the
    A. funds cannot be refunded
    B. funeral home selected cannot be changed
    C. merchandise and services selected cannot be changed
    D. funeral home must conduct the service for what funds are available

    3._____

4. A cause of death stated on a death certificate that indicates a failure of the heart is
    A. renal infarction
    B. diabetes mellitus
    C. cerebrovascular accident
    D. ventricular fibrillation

    4._____

5. When a decedent was not married and has no children, but has a will, which of the following does NOT have a right of final disposition?
    A. the state
    B. a parent
    C. a sibling
    D. personal representative of the estate

    5._____

6. When two or more persons enter into a contract with one or more other persons, the contract may be
   I. joint
   II. collective
   III. several
   IV. conditional

   A. I and III only
   B. I and IV only
   C. II and III only
   D. II and IV only

7. The Masonic Lodge performing at the graveside is an example of a
   A. more
   B. custom
   C. folkway
   D. ceremony

8. The "must behaviors" that indicate that an individual must abstain from certain acts are referred to as
   A. laws
   B. taboos
   C. culture
   D. folkways

9. In Maslow's Hierarchy of Needs, the lowest or basic need is
   A. esteem
   B. physiological need
   C. self-actualization
   D. belongingness and love

10. During a Roman Catholic funeral Mass, the casket for a lay person is usually placed
    A. parallel to the altar
    B. foot end toward the altar
    C. head end toward the altar
    D. in the narthex of the church

11. A practitioner arrives at a liturgical church for a service in which the processional and recessional will include clergy, casket bearers, casket and family. If the aisle is only wide enough to accommodate the casket, the casket bearers should
    A. walk in front of the casket behind the clergy
    B. walk alongside the casket
    C. walk between the casket and the family
    D. be seated in the last row of the church during the service

12. During a post-service conversation, the funeral director should advise families who want grief counseling to see a
    A. psychic
    B. psychologist
    C. preneed counselor
    D. physical therapist

13. An example of a softwood species casket would be
    A. oak
    B. pine
    C. cherry
    D. mahogany

14. The type of ledger that contains all of the accounts shown on the trial balance is known as a(n)
    A. audit ledger
    B. general ledger
    C. subsidiary ledger
    D. accounts receivable ledger

15. The funeral rite does which of the following?
    I. Completes the grieving process
    II. Honors the life that has been lived
    III. Provides a social function
    IV. Permits family and friends to call upon their faith and beliefs concerning the death

    A. I only
    B. II and III only
    C. II and IV only
    D. II, III and IV only

16. Written instruments drawn in a special form that can be transferred from person to person as a substitute for money or as an instrument of credit are known as
    A. fungibles
    B. bailments
    C. negotiable instruments
    D. certificates of deposit

17. Which of the following is NOT an interior style for a casket?
    A. crepe
    B. tufted
    C. shirred
    D. crushed

18. Johnson was engaged by Wilson to wash all the windows in Wilson's Funeral Home. Johnson was to be paid $500 and the job was to be completed within five days. Wilson was to have no control over the operation. Johnson is a(n)
    A. vendor
    B. agent of Wilson
    C. employee of Wilson
    D. independent contractor

19. Which of the following types of death would allow for anticipatory grief to occur?
    A. SIDS
    B. AIDS
    C. suicide
    D. homicide

20. The need for and the type of OSHA required employee training is determined by
    A. employee job description
    B. employee request for training
    C. funeral home training practices
    D. funeral home personnel training policy

21. How does a practitioner use the direct selection room procedure for vault selection?
    A. Leaving the selection room
    B. Remaining in the selection room
    C. Presenting photographs and leaving the room
    D. Sending the consumer to the vault manufacturer

22. The funeral rite satisfies all of the following needs of the survivors EXCEPT
    A. stress
    B. closure
    C. emotional
    D. psychological

23. What type of damages pay over and above the actual loss?
    A. Limited
    B. Nominal
    C. Punitive
    D. Compensatory

24. Which of the following is NOT specifically required by the Federal Trade Commission (FTC)?
    A. Casket Price List
    B. Funeral Agreement Form
    C. Outer Burial Container Price List
    D. Statement of Funeral Goods and Services Selected

25. The social values of the funeral rite are most commonly learned through   25._____
    A. religion
    B. education
    C. absorption
    D. enculturation

KEY (CORRECT ANSWERS)

1. A	11. B	21. A
2. A	12. B	22. B
3. D	13. B	23. C
4. D	14. B	24. C
5. A	15. D	25. A
6. A	16. C	
7. D	17. D	
8. B	18. D	
9. B	19. B	
10. B	20. C	

TEST 4

DIRECTIONS: Each question or incomplete statement is followed by several suggested answers or completions. Select the one that BEST answers the question or completes the statement. *PRINT THE LETTER OF THE CORRECT ANSWER IN THE SPACE AT THE RIGHT.*

1. According to merchandising guidelines, approximately how many caskets should be shown in a casket selection room?
    A. 6 minimum; 24 maximum
    B. 12 minimum; 24 maximum
    C. 12 minimum; 30 maximum
    D. 18 minimum; 30 maximum

    1._____

2. The party who assigns a contract is the
    A. agent
    B. bearer
    C. assignee
    D. assignor

    2._____

3. Wolfelt identifies which of the following as characteristics of stress?
    A. Focusing
    B. Long-term concentration
    C. Creativity and imagination
    D. Irritability and impatience

    3._____

4. Which of the following are input devices for a computer?
    I. mouse
    II. keyboard
    III. printer
    IV. monitor

    A. I and II only
    B. I, II and IV only
    C. II, III and IV only
    D. I, II, III and IV

    4._____

5. During the Dark Ages, a Christian burial in a church graveyard was denied for
    A. suicides
    B. divorcees
    C. widowers
    D. drunkards

    5._____

6. Within an extended patriarchal family, who would assume control of the family at the death of the father?
    A. Tom, son, age 37
    B. Steve, son, age 32
    C. Deborah, mother, age 58
    D. Jake, mother's brother, age 54

    6._____

7. What is the PRIMARY function of word-processing software?
   A. Producing graphic presentations
   B. Producing written documents
   C. Listing, calculating and sorting data
   D. Storing information in a data file cabinet

8. Consideration in a contract could be
   I. personal property
   II. money
   III. a promise of service
   IV. a promise to refrain from doing an illegal act

   A. II only
   B. I and IV only
   C. I, II and III only
   D. I, II, III and IV

9. The Fair Labor Standards Act covers which of the following areas of employment law?
   I. Minimum wage requirement
   II. Overtime compensation
   III. Equal pay
   IV. Reasonable accommodations

   A. I, II and III only
   B. I, II and IV only
   C. I, III and IV only
   D. I and II only

10. Compared to the extended (joint) family, a nuclear family is
    A. less mobile
    B. generally more liberal in thought
    C. generally the larger family system
    D. less dependent on employment outside the home

11. Variable costs, amount of workmanship involved and species availability are
    A. advantages of wood over metal caskets
    B. disadvantages of wood over metal caskets
    C. reasons why hardwood caskets may cost more than metal caskets
    D. factors that do not make each wood casket individual and unique

12. The record listing the merchandise and supplies on hand at any given time is called
    A. a ledger
    B. a journal
    C. inventory
    D. itemization

13. The increments between casket prices, when arranged in order of their increasing value, is called
    A. indexing
    B. regression
    C. progression
    D. quartiling

14. When placing floral arrangements next to the casket, the funeral director should place
    A. flowers as they come in
    B. family flowers in the foyer
    C. family flower nearest the casket
    D. the same color of flowers together

15. Which of the following are associated with filing suit in a civil action?
    I. Discovery
    II. Process
    III. Petition
    IV. Answer

    A. I and II only
    B. I, III and IV only
    C. II, III and IV only
    D. I, II, III and IV

16. The death of a child would likely be felt more within the _____ family.
    A. joint
    B. nuclear
    C. generational
    D. modified extended nuclear

17. Aftercare programs have come into being because of the
    A. decrease in psychotherapy
    B. increase in social support
    C. absence of clear social norms
    D. staying power of the family unit

18. The first step to the Americans with Disabilities Act (ADA) compliance is the creation of a
    A. priority list
    B. needs assessment
    C. compliance statement
    D. written compliance plan

19. Another name for client-centered counseling is
    A. directive
    B. expeditious
    C. nondirective
    D. psychoanalytical

4 (#4)

20. A synonym for vestibule is   20._____
    A. sanctuary   B. chancel
    C. narthex   D. nave

KEY (CORRECT ANSWERS)

1. A	11. C
2. D	12. C
3. D	13. C
4. A	14. C
5. A	15. C
6. D	16. B
7. B	17. C
8. C	18. B
9. A	19. C
10. A	20. C

TEST 5

DIRECTIONS: Each question or incomplete statement is followed by several suggested answers or completions. Select the one that BEST answers the question or completes the statement. *PRINT THE LETTER OF THE CORRECT ANSWER IN THE SPACE AT THE RIGHT.*

1. A child at a viewing clings to one of the adults. When asked by the practitioner what is wrong, the child says that the deceased is going to jump out of the casket and get the child. According to Grollman, the age of this child based upon the understanding of death is ____ years.
   A. 1-4   B. 5-9   C. 10-14   D. 15-19

   1._____

2. The restatement of an adult's willingness to be bound by a promise made during minority is known as
   A. voidable   B. rescindment
   C. ratification   D. null and void

   2._____

3. Which of the following accounts normally has a credit balance?
   A. asset   B. expense
   C. liability   D. prepaid expense

   3._____

4. A widow states, "I just can't wait to move out of the house because everything reminds me of my husband. It will be better for my children too." Which of the following grief concepts does this individual NOT understand?
   A. Moving unties emotional bonds
   B. Moving helps the grief process
   C. There are no geographical escapes from memories
   D. Children do better when they are removed from memories

   4._____

5. An abnormal fear of death is called
   A. regression   B. necrophilia
   C. thanatology   D. thanatophobia

   5._____

6. Religion is defined as a culturally entrenched pattern of behavior made up of
   I. sacred beliefs
   II. emotional feelings accompanying beliefs
   III. overt conduct implementing beliefs
   IV. universally accepted beliefs

   A. I, II and III only
   B. I, II and IV only
   C. I, III and IV only
   D. II, III and IV only

   6._____

7. The only fee permitted by the Federal Trade Commission (FTC) to be nondeclinable at the outset of the funeral transaction is the charge for
    A. embalming
    B. use of vehicles
    C. use of facilities
    D. basic services for funeral director and staff for overhead

7._____

8. Chromium is added to carbon steel primarily to
    A. make it shinier
    B. reduce the cost of production
    C. increase the resistance to rust and corrosion
    D. eliminate the need for a thicker/stronger product

8._____

9. Lindemann identified which of the following characteristics of grief?
    I. Somatic distress
    II. Clinical depression
    III. Preoccupation with images of the deceased
    IV. Hostile reactions

    A. I and IV only
    B. II and III only
    C. I, III and IV only
    D. II, III and IV only

9._____

10. Which of the following is an example of a signed agreement of an oral understanding?
    A. Music selections
    B. Embalming authorization
    C. Types of flowers
    D. Request for military honors

10._____

11. A practitioner serves a family and provides both services and merchandise. The state requires the funeral home to pay 4% sales tax on merchandise. Prices are as follows:
    Services $2,000
    Casket $2,250
    Vault $1,600
    TOTAL $5,850
    How much sales tax does the funeral director pay the state?
    A. $80   B. $90   C. $154   D. $234

11._____

12. A helpful relationship in which one party seeks to facilitate the development of informed choices and meaningful actions at a critical time within the context of another's life is
    A. friendship   B. counseling
    C. therapy   D. crisis

12._____

13. Gross sales minus sales returns and allowances and minus discounts on sales yields
    A. net sales
    B. gross profit
    C. total purchases
    D. cost of merchandise sold

14. Blame perceived to be directed at one's self by others is the definition of
    A. anger
    B. shame
    C. frustration
    D. helplessness

15. Which of the following is NOT a characteristic of a general partnership?
    A. Limited life
    B. Limited liability
    C. Participation of income
    D. Co-ownership of property

16. A funeral rite that is adjusted to the needs and wants of those directly involved and to the trends of the times is called
    A. adaptive
    B. humanistic
    C. traditional
    D. a memorial service

17. If an individual was intoxicated when the contractual portion of the Statement of Funeral Goods and Services Selected was signed, the contract is
    A. void
    B. valid
    C. voidable
    D. unenforceable

18. Which of the following is primarily liable on a promissory note?
    A. maker
    B. payee
    C. endorser
    D. endorsee

19. The Jewish term for the ceremony of washing the deceased before burial is
    A. Tallith
    B. Taharah
    C. Tehilim
    D. Tachrichim

20. Which of the following is part of a computer's CPU?
    A. Monitor
    B. Keyboard
    C. Disk drive
    D. Memory chip

KEY (CORRECT ANSWERS)

1. B	11. C
2. C	12. B
3. C	13. A
4. C	14. B
5. D	15. B
6. C	16. B
7. D	17. C
8. C	18. A
9. C	19. B
10. B	20. D

EXAMINATION SECTION

TEST 1

DIRECTIONS: Each question or incomplete statement is followed by several suggested answers or completions. Select the one that BEST answers the question or completes the statement. *PRINT THE LETTER OF THE CORRECT ANSWER IN THE SPACE AT THE RIGHT.*

1. Which enzyme allows *Staphylococcus aureus* to penetrate the body's connective tissues permitting easy spread of infection throughout the body?
   A. Coagulase
   B. Lipase
   C. Hyaluronidase
   D. Esterase

   1.____

2. A _____ is a genus of bacteria having a flexible cell wall but no flagella in the traditional sense. Movement in these organisms occurs by contractions of long filaments that run the length of the cell wall.
   A. sarcinae   B. spirochete   C. protozoa   D. prion

   2.____

3. Which of the following is a small proteinaceous infectious agent which almost certainly does not have a nucleic acid genome and, therefore, resists inactivation by procedures that modify nucleic acids?
   A. Streptococci   B. Prions   C. Parasites   D. Saprophytes

   3.____

4. _____ is a genus of spiral bacteria which are curved or bent rods that resemble commas.
   A. Vibrio   B. Spirillum   C. Spirochete   D. Streptobacilli

   4.____

5. A _____ is one of a group of minute infectious agents with certain exceptions not resolved in the light microscope and characterized by lack of independent metabolism and by the ability to replicate only within living cell hosts.
   A. vibrio   B. virus   C. prion   D. bacteria

   5.____

6. Which of the following is defined as dilution or weakening of virulence of a microorganism, thus reducing or abolishing pathogenicity?
   A. Antisepsis   B. Antagonism   C. Virucide   D. Attenuation

   6.____

7. Which of the following is the causative agent of generalized decomposition?
   A. *Bacillus anthracis*
   B. *Neisseria meningitides*
   C. *Proteus vulgaris*
   D. *Escherichia coli*

   7.____

8. A _____ is defined as an inflamed, swollen, or enlarged lymph node exhibiting suppuration, occurring commonly after infective disease due to absorption of infected material.
   A. bubo   B. vibrio   C. prion   D. eschar

   8.____

101

9. Which of the following is the causative agent of tissue gas?
   A. *Clostridium tetani*   B. *Clostridium perfringens*
   C. *Mycobacterium avium*   D. *Yersinia pestis*

10. Who was the FIRST person to advocate aseptic practices/treatment to minimize fatalities?
    A. Edward Jenner   B. Joseph Lister
    C. Robert Hooke   D. Rudolph Virchow

11. Which of the following refers to a disease that occurs continuously in a particular region but has low mortality?
    A. Pandemic   B. Epidemic   C. Endemic   D. Transdemic

12. A facultative _____ is an organism that prefers an oxygen environment but is capable of living and growing in its absence.
    A. aerobe   B. anaerobe   C. saprophyte   D. parasite

13. A facultative _____ is an organism that prefers organic matter as a source of nutrition but can adapt to the use of dead organic matter under certain conditions.
    A. aerobe   B. anaerobe   C. saprophyte   D. parasite

14. Which of the following is defined as an interactive relationship between two organisms in which one is harmed and the other benefits?
    A. Parasitism   B. Mutualism
    C. Communalism   D. Synergism

15. A strict _____ is a microbe that can only live in the presence of free oxygen.
    A. aerobe   B. anaerobe   B. saprophyte   D. parasite

16. A strict _____ is an organism that is completely dependent on its living host for survival.
    A. aerobe   B. anaerobe   C. saprophyte   D. parasite

17. Which of the following, also known as immunoglobulin, is a glycoprotein substance developed by the body in response to, and interacting specifically with, an antigen?
    A. Fomite   B. Antibody   C. Mesophile   D. Toxin

18. _____ are bacteria that thrive best at high temperatures between 40°C and 70°C.
    A. Mesophiles   B. Thermophiles
    C. Iodophores   D. Psychrophiles

19. Which of the following is a genus of gram-positive, non-motile, opportunistic bacteria which tend to aggregate in irregular, grape-like clusters?
    A. Streptococcus   B. Meningococcus
    C. Gonococcus   D. Staphylococcus

20. A(n) _____ is an organism that exists as part of normal flora but can become pathogenic under certain conditions.
    A. parasite   B. opportunist   C. antagonist   D. protagonist

21. A microorganism that requires very little free oxygen is referred to as
    A. aerobic
    B. anaerobic
    C. microaerophilic
    D. microaerophobic

22. Which of the following is known to inhabit the nose, therefore embalmers should be watchful for airborne transmission as well as direct contact with the nose?
    A. Streptococcus
    B. Gonococcus
    C. Meningococcus
    D. Staphylococcus

23. Lobar pneumonia, pneumococcal meningitis, and otitis media are three conditions of clinical importance to embalmers and are all caused by
    A. streptococcus
    B. gonococcus
    C. meningococcus
    D. staphylococcus

24. Which of the following is a gram-positive, spore-forming anaerobe that produces two endotoxins, is found in enterics, and is shed in the feces?
    A. *Clostridium tetani*
    B. *Clostridium perfringens*
    C. *Clostridium botulinum*
    D. *Clostridium difficile*

25. _____ is a gram-positive, encapsulated, high virulent diplococcus in which 70% of the population are healthy carriers and most cases occur in individuals between 1 month and 4 years of age.
    A. Pneumococcal meningitis
    B. Streptococcal pyrogens
    C. Puerperal sepsis
    D. Rheumatic fever

KEY (CORRECT ANSWERS)

1.	C	11.	C
2.	B	12.	B
3.	B	13.	C
4.	A	14.	A
5.	B	15.	A
6.	D	16.	D
7.	C	17.	B
8.	A	18.	B
9.	B	19.	D
10.	B	20.	B

21. C
22. D
23. A
24. D
25. A

TEST 2

DIRECTIONS: Each question or incomplete statement is followed by several suggested answers or completions. Select the one that BEST answers the question or completes the statement. *PRINT THE LETTER OF THE CORRECT ANSWER IN THE SPACE AT THE RIGHT.*

1. An _____ is an organic compound containing one or more hydroxyl (-OH) groups. The general formula is R-OH where R is a hydrocarbon group.
    A. alcohol   B. aldehyde   C. alkane   D. alkene

    1.____

2. Which of the following, illustrated in the image shown at the right, is an unsaturated hydrocarbon containing a double bond?
    A. Alkane   B. Alkene   C. Alkyne   D. Alkyl

    $H-C \equiv C-(CH_2)_n-H$

    2.____

3. Any compound that can act as both an acid and a base in solution is said to be
    A. ampotheric
    B. hydrospheric
    C. lithospheric
    D. ionospheric

    3.____

4. Which of the following is a solution-like system in which the size of the solute particle is between 1 and 100 nanometers and the particles of solute pass through filters not membranes?
    A. Suspension   B. Colloid   C. Emulsion   D. Tincture

    4.____

5. A(n) _____ is a subatomic particle with a negative electrical charge and a mass that is found outside the nucleus of an atom.
    A. neutron   B. electron   C. positron   D. prion

    5.____

6. A(n) _____ is a mixture of two insoluble liquids, one being dispersed throughout the other in small droplets.
    A. suspension   B. colloid   C. emulsion   D. tincture

    6.____

7. Which of the following is the branch of chemistry that studies the properties and reactions of elements, excluding organic or certain carbon containing compounds?
    A. Biochemistry
    B. Inorganic chemistry
    C. Physical chemistry
    D. Analytical chemistry

    7.____

8. Which of the following is the process of swelling and softening of tissues and organs as a result of absorbing moisture?
    A. Imbibition
    B. Saponification
    C. Emulsification
    D. Engorgement

    8.____

9. Which of the following, as illustrated in the image shown at the right, is an organic compound containing nitrogen or any compounds formed from ammonia by replacement of one or more hydrogen atoms by organic radicals?
   A. Amino acid
   B. Amide
   C. Amine
   D. Alkyl group

10. _____ is the reaction between a fat and a strong base to produce glycerol and the salt of a fatty acid.
    A. Putrefaction
    B. Saponification
    C. Fermentation
    D. Decarboxylation

11. Which of the following is the process of the decomposition of proteins by the actions of enzymes from anaerobic bacteria?
    A. Sublimation
    B. Putrefaction
    C. Imbibition
    D. Denaturation

12. Which of the following, illustrated in the image shown at the right, is a chemical compound similar to alcohol in which the oxygen of the hydroxyl group is replaced by a sulfhydral group?
    A. Urotropin
    B. Mercaptan
    C. Protein
    D. Isomer

13. Which of the following is the product of the neutralization reaction between formaldehyde and ammonia?
    A. Tryptophan   B. Mercaptan   C. Urotropin   D. Glycogen

14. _____ is the study of the physical and chemical changes of the human body that results from the process of death.
    A. Biochemistry
    B. Embalming chemistry
    C. Thanatochemistry
    D. Organic chemistry

15. _____ is added to inhibit polymerization when formaldehyde is dissolved in water.
    A. Glycol   B. Methanol   C. Atenolol   D. Metoprolol

16. Which of the following refers to the type of chemical reaction that involves the removal of oxygen from inorganic substances?
    A. Oxidation
    B. Decarboxylation
    C. Reduction
    D. Induction

17. Paraform exists at room temperature in a _____ state. 17.____
    A. solid   B. liquid   C. gaseous   D. super-solid

18. _____ alcohol is another name for Methanol. 18.____
    A. Wood   B. Grain   C. Butyl   D. Propyl

19. Which of the following would be the result of partial oxidation of CH_2O? 19.____
    A. Methanol
    B. Methene
    C. Methane
    D. Methanoic acid

20. _____ would be an example of a dialdehyde. 20.____
    A. Formaldehyde
    B. Glutaraldehyde
    C. Acetaldehyde
    D. Benzaldehyde

21. A(n) _____ solution would result in the hemolysis of red blood cells. 21.____
    A. neutral   B. hypertonic   C. hypotonic   D. isotonic

22. Where are the valence electrons affecting metallic and non-metallic compounds located? 22.____
    A. Nucleus of the atom
    B. Inner orbital ring
    C. Outer orbital ring
    C. Intraorbital ring

23. _____ is defined as the contraction of a cell after exposure to a hypertonic solution due to loss of water through osmosis. 23.____
    A. Crenation
    B. Putrefaction
    C. Imbibition
    D. Denaturation

24. A(n) _____ bond occurs between carbon to carbon in an organic compound. 24.____
    A. peptide
    B. ionic
    C. covalent
    D. polar covalent

25. Which of the following is an example of a disaccharide? 25.____
    A. Sucrose   B. Glucose   C. Cellulose   D. Fructose

KEY (CORRECT ANSWERS)

1.	A	11.	B
2.	C	12.	B
3.	A	13.	C
4.	B	14.	C
5.	B	15.	B
6.	C	16.	C
7.	B	17.	A
8.	A	18.	A
9.	C	19.	D
10.	B	20.	B

21. D
22. C
23. A
24. C
25. A

TEST 3

DIRECTIONS: Each question or incomplete statement is followed by several suggested answers or completions. Select the one that BEST answers the question or completes the statement. *PRINT THE LETTER OF THE CORRECT ANSWER IN THE SPACE AT THE RIGHT.*

1. Which of the following refers to a general state of ill health, often associated with emaciation?
   A. Anasarca   B. Aplasia   C. Cachexia   D. Atrophy

   1.____

2. _____ is the condition in which the descent of a testis into the scrotum is stopped at some point in its normal path.
   A. Cretinism
   B. Cryptorchidism
   C. Priapism
   D. Embolism

   2.____

3. _____ gangrene is a condition that results when the body part that dies has had little blood flow and remains aseptic. Commonly occurs when the arteries are obstructed.
   A. Dry   B. Wet   C. Gas   D. Fournier

   3.____

4. _____ is defined as fluid or cellular debris exuding from blood vessels and deposited in tissues or tissue surfaces, usually as a result of inflammation.
   A. Epistaxis
   B. Exsanguination
   C. Exacerbation
   D. Exudate

   4.____

5. A goiter is an abnormal enlargement of the thyroid gland due to deficiency of
   A. calcium   B. sodium   C. iodine   D. potassium

   5.____

6. Which of the following refers to the condition of blood in the sputum?
   A. Hematemesis
   B. Hematuria
   C. Hemophilia
   D. Hemoptysis

   6.____

7. Which of the following is defined as an increase in the size of an organ or part due to excessive but regulated growth?
   A. Hyperplasia
   B. Hypertrophy
   C. Organomegaly
   D. Hyperemia

   7.____

8. If a disease or medical condition is the result of an unknown cause, the condition is said to be
   A. homeopathic
   B. naturopathic
   C. idiopathic
   D. osteopathic

   8.____

9. Which of the following refers to the process of seepage of diffusion into the tissue of substances that are not ordinarily present?
   A. Infection
   B. Infestation
   C. Infiltration
   D. Inflammation

   9.____

10. _____ is the study of disease to ascertain cause and manner of death.
    A. Forensic Pathology B. Microscopic Pathology
    C. Macroscopic Pathology D. Histopathology

11. Which of the following is a disease marked by softening of the bones due to faulty calcification in adulthood?
    A. Osteopenia B. Osteomalacia
    C. Osteomyelitis D. Osteoporosis

12. Which of the following is defined as antemortem, extravascular, pinpoint blood discolorations that are visible as purple-blue hemorrhages under the skin?
    A. Ecchymosis B. Phocomelia C. Petechiae D. Purpura

13. _____ is a lung disorder caused by inhaling mineral dust where the person can inhale but cannot exhale properly.
    A. Tuberculosis B. Emphysema
    C. Pneumonia D. Pneumoconiosis

14. _____ transmission occurs when an insect carries a pathogen from the source and deposits the pathogen on the potential host.
    A. Biological B. Mechanical C. Zoonotic D. Autosomal

15. In what organ does fat necrosis most often occur?
    A. Liver B. Spleen C. Pancreas D. Gallbladder

16. Anthracosis is a medical condition caused from the shortage of what kind of particles in the lung and regional lymph nodes?
    A. Carbon B. Silicone C. Asbestos D. Wood

17. Which of the following is described as a marked decrease in blood carbon dioxide content?
    A. Abatement B. Acidosis C. Alkalosis D. Acapnia

18. _____ is defined as a loss of consciousness from deficient oxygen.
    A. Anoxia B. Asphyxia C. Anasarca D. Acapnia

19. Which of the following is the green pigment in the bile?
    A. Bilirubin B. Biliverdin C. Phycobilin D. Stercobilin

20. Any disease that is caused by the medical profession is said to be`
    A. pathogenic B. Iatrogenic C. teratogenic D. xenogenic

21. Which of the following refers to any foreign or heterogeneous substance contained in a cell or in any tissue or organ that was not introduced as a result of trauma?
    A. Inclusion B. Infarction C. Infestation D. Infiltration

22. Which of the following is defined as the ratio of sick to well in a community?
    A. Mortality rate
    B. Morbidity rate
    C. Prevalence
    D. Occurrence

23. A condition in which the endometrial tissue is located elsewhere is referred to as
    A. oophoritis
    B. salpingitis
    C. endocervicitis
    D. endometriosis

24. Which of the following medical conditions cause overproduction of bone in the skull, vertebrae, and pelvis?
    A. Acromegaly
    B. Osteosarcoma
    C. Paget's Disease
    D. Osteochondritis

25. Which of the following is defined as hyperadrenalism and is manifested by a characteristic bronzing of the skin?
    A. Cushing's Disease
    B. Waterhouse-Friderichsen Syndrome
    C. Addison's Disease
    D. Wilson's Disease

KEY (CORRECT ANSWERS)

1.	C	11.	B
2.	B	12.	C
3.	A	13.	D
4.	D	14.	B
5.	C	15.	C
6.	D	16.	A
7.	A	17.	D
8.	C	18.	B
9.	C	19.	B
10.	A	20.	B

21.	A
22.	B
23.	D
24.	C
25.	C

TEST 4

DIRECTIONS: Each question or incomplete statement is followed by several suggested answers or completions. Select the one that BEST answers the question or completes the statement. *PRINT THE LETTER OF THE CORRECT ANSWER IN THE SPACE AT THE RIGHT.*

1. Which of the following is a series of membranes that form canals which transport nutrients and other materials through the cell?
    A. Cytoplasm
    B. Ribosomes
    C. Mitochondria
    D. Endoplasmic reticulum

    1.____

2. The _____ artery bifurcates into the right subclavian and right common carotid arteries.
    A. brachiocephalic
    B. axillary
    C. subclavian
    D. ulnar

    2.____

3. The union of the splenic vein and the superior mesenteric vein forms the _____ vein.
    A. inferior mesenteric
    B. portal
    C. left gastroomental
    D. left colic

    3.____

4. The liver receives its blood supply from which of the following blood vessels?
    A. Left gastric artery
    B. Common hepatic artery
    C. Celiac trunk artery
    D. Superior mesenteric artery

    4.____

5. What heart valve is located in the right atrio-ventricular septum?
    A. Mitral valve
    B. Bicuspid valve
    C. Tricuspid valve
    D. Pulmonary semilunar valve

    5.____

6. What portion of the skull is removed during a cranial autopsy?
    A. Occipital bone
    B. Calvarium
    C. Temporal bone
    D. Zygomatic bone

    6.____

7. What organ is located in a retroperitoneal position?
    A. Liver   B. Stomach   C. Spleen   D. Kidney

    7.____

8. Which of the following is the unpaired artery associated with the Circle of Willis?
    A. Internal carotid artery
    B. Anterior cerebral artery
    C. Posterior communicating artery
    D. Basilar artery

    8.____

9. Which of the following, also referred to as the "Little Vinegar Cup," is the socket of the hip joint?
    A. Acetabulum
    B. Ilium
    C. Ischium
    D. Cox

    9.____

10. The _____ is located just behind the external acoustic meatus and lateral to the styloid process to provide a point of attachment for the digastric and sternocleidomastoid muscles.
    A. temporomandibular joint
    B. mastoid process
    C. pterion
    D. external occipital protuberance

11. Which of the following is an inferior branch of the subclavian arteries that provide collateral circulation to the legs?
    A. Internal mammary arteries
    B. Vertebral arteries
    C. Inferior vena cava
    D. Musculophrenic arteries

12. The _____ forms at L5 with the caval opening into the thoracic cavity at T8.
    A. superior vena cava
    B. inferior vena cava
    C. superior mesenteric artery
    D. inferior mesenteric artery

13. The _____ artery begins at the 2nd right costal cartilage and ends at the upper border of the 2nd right sternoclavicular articulation.
    A. right coronary
    B. right common carotid
    C. right subclavian
    D. innominate

14. The _____ artery begins at the level of the 2nd costal cartilage and ends at the superior border of the thyroid cartilage.
    A. right common carotid
    B. left common carotid
    C. right subclavian
    D. left subclavian

15. Which of the following begins at the lateral border of the first rib and extends to the inferior border of the tendon of teres major muscle and is located behind the medial border of the coracobrachialis muscle?
    A. Right subclavian artery
    B. Right vertebral artery
    C. Right axillary artery
    D. Right internal mammary artery

16. Which of the following, illustrated by the image shown at the right, is a thin trapezoidal bone of the skull forming the posterior and inferior parts of the nasal septum?
    A. Maxilla
    B. Vomer bone
    C. Sphenoid bone
    D. Zygomatic bone

17. The galea aponeurotica is the tendon of which of the following muscles?
    A. Occipitofrontalis muscle
    B. Levator labi muscle
    C. Oribicularis oculi muscle
    D. Masseter muscle

18. Which of the following is a ring of muscle that guards the opening between the stomach and the duodenum?
    A. Lower esophageal sphincter
    B. Ileocecal sphincter
    C. Pyloric sphincter
    D. Precapillary sphincter

19. The milk-like liquid composed of lymph and globules of digested fats coursing through the lacteals during digestion is called
    A. bile
    B. chyle
    C. serum
    D. plasma

20. Which of the following refers to an air cavity within a bone, often referred to as a sinus?
    A. Antrum
    B. Meatus
    C. Condyle
    D. Fissure

21. Which of the following refers to a temporarily unossified area between the cranial bones of an infant?
    A. Fissure
    B. Fontanel
    C. Foramen
    D. Fossa

22. The ____ muscle, also known as the diaphragm, separates the thorax from the abdomen and contains passageways for veins, arteries, and nerves.
    A. sternocleidomastoid
    B. internal intercostal
    C. phrenic
    D. internal oblique

23. What structure represents the lateral border of the femoral triangle?
    A. Inguinal ligament
    B. Adductor longus muscle
    C. Sartorius muscle
    D. Latissimus dorsi muscle

24. Which of the following is defined as fluid secreted by the peritoneum which lubricates the organs and reduces the friction when the organs slide against each other?
    A. Bile
    B. Chyle
    C. Serum
    D. Plasma

25. Which of the following, illustrated in the red portion of the image shown at the right, is the first section of the large intestine where the small intestine meets the large intestine?
    A. Jejunum
    B. Cecum
    C. Ascending colon
    D. Sigmoid colon

KEY (CORRECT ANSWERS)

1. D
2. A
3. B
4. C
5. C

6. B
7. D
8. D
9. A
10. B

11. A
12. B
13. D
14. B
15. C

16. B
17. A
18. C
19. B
20. A

21. B
22. C
23. C
24. C
25. B

BASIC FUNDAMENTALS OF FUNERAL SERVICE SCIENCE

I EMBALMING

    A. Orientation and Introduction
General - definition of embalming, summary of embalming process; need for embalming; history of embalming; professional and ethical conduct-moral consideraton; legal considerations; sanitation - personal and environmental hygiene.

    B. Death
Definition; terms associated; types of death; tests for death.

    C. Pre-Embalming Changes
Antemortem (agonal changes); postmortem.

    D. Technical Orientation of Embalming
Equipment, instruments and accessory materials; pre-embalming analysis; position of body (prior to embalming); posing the feature; eye enucleation restoration.

    E. Selection of arteries
Definitions - linear guide, anatomical guide, anatomical limits; arteries most commonly used in embalming; factors goerning selection of artery to be injected on any given body; proper technique for raising vessels; types of sutures for closing incisions; other methods of closing incision.

    F. Injection
Methods of creating fluid pressure; pressure discussion - definition, Injection pressure (factors affecting, recommended pressures, procedure), rate of flow.

    G. Types of Embalming Chemicals
Arterial -function, purpose, classification, components, effects on body tissues and tissue fluids and proteins; cavity - puruose, dilutiens, composition, supplemental fluids - pre-injection, co-injection, homectant special arterial fluids, high index fluids; accessory chemicals-hardening compounds; mold preventive agents, preservative powders, cealing agents, pack applications; safety in handling embalming chemicals.

    H. Dilution, Distribution, Diffusion
Primary; secondary; fluid distribution, fluid diffusion; signs of fluid distribution and diffusion.

    I. Drainage
Purpose and importance; drainage technique - veins; methods of drainage in relation to injection; methods of stimulating.

    J. Cavity Treatment
Definition, purpose, abdominal regions-four region plan; trocar guides; aspiration and injection equipment and methods; materials to be aspirated purge.

K. Autopsies, Necropsies or Postmortem Examinations
Regional - cranial, thoracic and/or abdominal autopsy, spinal autopsy; exploratory.

L. Postmortem Conditions and Their Embalming Treatments
Discolorations; vascular difficulties; decompositon; dehydration; body fluid accumulation; purge; deformities and malformations, contagion and infection; radiation.

II RESTORATIVE ART

A. Orientation
Definitions - restorative art, pysiognomy; restoratins for which permission is not sought; real and complimentary charges for restoration.

B. Surface Bones of the Cranium
Geometric form of normal scull-oval from three views; external cranial bones.

C. Surface Bones of the Face
External facial bones-location, surfaces.

D. Priminences, Depressions and Cavities
Description and location of prominences, cavities and depressions.

E. Facial Proportions
Values in order to make comparisons with photograph; horizontal lines (imaginary), vertical lines (imaginary) porportional relationships based on horizontal and vertical lines; additional measurements.

F. Reference to the Photograph
Comparative values of snapshots and professional portraits; values of the 3/4 view photo; value of profile view; definition of highlights and shadows.

G. Facial Profiles
Basic linear forms (disregarding nasal profile); combinations of basic linear forms; most common form; least common form.

H. Head forms (Frontal View)
Geometric forms described; most common form; least common form.

I. Bilateral Forms of the Head and Features
Definition; asymmetry of paired structures; surfaces exhibiting a similarity of bilateral curvature; methods of comparing bilateral curvatures during a wax restoration.

J. Identifying Facial Markings (Cause by Muscles)
Factors responsible for facial marking; definitions-furrow, groove fold (eminence); reproduction of furrows, grooves and folds on wax area, classification of facial markings; definitions and examples of natural facial markings and acquired facial markings.

K. Wax Modeling
    Wages-types, qualifications of satisfactory waxes, cosmetics (in, under and upon wax), softening wax; conditions of deep and surface tissues necesary for wax restoration (and methods and materials used); technique of reproducing surface detail and contour; techniques of modeling features.

L. Structures of the Ear (Pinna)
    General characteristics; anatomical guides for locating ear; description of ear structures.

M. Structures of the Nose
    General Description-racial classifications, profile classifications; anatomy, parts of the nose; nose restoration- physical and medical distortion.

N. Structures of the Mouth
    Characteristics; identification of mouth parts, location and type of Facial markings; description of structures of structures; cosmetic application to alter thickness and width, restoratins of mouth.

O. Structures of the Closed Eye
    Profile forms;line of closure, size and form of eyelids; location and description of fossa, supraorbital area, inner canthus sulci; linear sulci, cilia; supercilium, eye restorations, separated eyelids, orbital pouch, dehydrated inner canthus.

P. General Restorative Treatments
    Classificatin of cases requiring restorative art treatment; abrasions and lacerations; bleaching; burns; cancer treatment; decapitation; distensions; desquamation; excisions; fractures; hair restoration.

Q. Death Masks
    Differentiation between negative (mild) and positive (cast); methods of hastening and of retarding setting time of Plaster of Paris.

R. Definition of color; the spectrum;absorption and reflection in naming colors; measures of color; pigment theory (Rang System); color schemes; efect of colored lights on colored objects.

S. Cosmetology
    Coloring methods; pigments of the skin; pigment cosmetics necessary to match the skin; types of complexions; methods of applying external complexion compounds; change of overtones on an applied cosmetic; highlights and shadows, natural warm-color areas on face and hands; natural color of lips; changing dimensions of lips; effect of powder; treatment of complete (or extensive) discoloration.

III MICROBIOLOGY

    A. Orientation
Definition of microbiology, microorganisms; divisions of microbiology; microorganisms of major health importance.

    B. Anatomy of Bacteria
Morphology of bacteria; structure of bacteria.

    C. Physiology of Bacteria
Reproduction, definition of bacterial colony; conditions affecting bacterial growth.

    D. Control of Microorganisms
Definitions-sterilization, disinfection, disinfectant, germicide (bactericide, fungicide, viricide), insecticide, bacteriostasis, fumigation; physical methods of control; chemical methods of control-desirable qualities of an ideal disinfectant, factors influencing action of disinfectants, description of disinfectants suitable for mortuary prodecures.

    E. Microorganisms and Disease
Definitions-infection, pathogenic organisms, contamination, infestation, virulence, elective localizatin;types of infections; toxic products of pathogenic bacterial; sources of infection; modes of transmission of infections; portals of entry of pathogens; methods of exit of the pathogens, factors influencing occurrence of an infection; defenses of doby against infection.

    F. Immunology
Antigens, examples; antibodies, examples; kinds of immunity; comparison of humoral and cell mediated immunity; hypersensitivity; AIDS.

    G. Specific Bacteria and Infections Pathogenicity, portals of entry and exit, modes of transmission of: staphylococcus aureua, streptococcus pneumoniae, neisseria gonorrhoeae, neisseria meningitidis, clostridium tenani, clostricium perfringens, corynebacterium diphtheriae, salmonella enteriditis, francisella tularensis, mycobacterium tuberculosis; treponema pallidum, other bacteria and diseases-vibrio comma, yersinia pestis, klebsiella pneumoniae, clostricium botulinum, bacillus anthracis, leptospira interrogans, hemophilus influenzae, bacteroides sp., proteus sp., pseudomonas sp.

    H. Rickettsia
Definition; general characteristics; important ricket-tsial diseases.

    I. Viruses
Definition; important viral diseases.

    J. Chlamydia
Definition, important diseases.

    K. Pathogenic Protozoa
Definition of protozoa.

IV PATHOLOGY

    A. Introduction
Definitions-pathology, general pathology, special pathology; divisions of pathology; importance of autopsy as tool in advancement of medical science; attitude of funeral director toward autopsies.

    B. Disease - General
Nature of disease-definition of disease, relation of cellular changes to disease, descriptive terminology relating to disease, causes of disease.

    C. Cellular Reaction to Injury
Types of regressive cellular changes.

    D. Inflammation and Repair
Definition of inflammation; function of inflammation; process of inflammation and repair; types of inflammation; repair.

    E. Disturbances in Circulation
Edema; hyperemia; ischemia; thrombosis; embolism; infarction; hemorrhage and terms relating to hemorrage, definition circulatory shock.

    F. Infectious Diseases
Communicable diseases-streptococcal infections, staphylococcal infections, intestinal infections, infections with major effects caused by exotoxins, tuberculosis, venereal diseases.

    G. Tumors and Cysts Neoplasms.

    H. Diseases of the Blood
Reactive changes; anemia; hematopoietic disorders; bleeding disorders.

    I. Diseases of the Heart and Blood Vessels
Definitions and causes of diseases of the heart and blood vessels.

    J. Diseases of the Digestive System
Definitions and causes of diseases of digestive organs; peritonitis.

    K. Diseases of the Respiratory System
Definitions and causes of diseases of the respiratory organs.

    L. Diseases of the Urinary Tract
Definitions of diseases of the urinary tract; uremia; kidney diseases structure of the ureters and urethra.

    M. Diseases of the Nervous System.
Trauma; meningitis; cerebrovascular accident; definitions of hydrocephalus encephalitis, cerebral abscess, general paresis, myelitis, poliomyelitis, neuritis, epilepsy.

N. Diseases of Female Reproductive System
Definitions and causes of diseases of the uterus, fallopian tubes; ovaries, vagina.

O. Diseases of Male Reproductive System
Definitions and diseases of testis, epididymis; prostatitis; diseases of the scrotum.

P. Diseases of Bones and Joints
Definitions and diseases of the bones and joints.

Q. Diseases of Endocrine Glands
Definitions of endocrine gland diseases; diabetes mellitus compliations.

FORENSIC (MEDICO-LEGAL) PATHOLOGY

R. Coroner and Medical Examiner
Jurisdiction, qualification, inquest.

S. Medico-legal Investigation
Types of death with medico-legal potential, determination of jurisdiction medical examiner's case, purpose of ordinary autopsy versus aims of forensic autopsy.

T. Injuries: General Features
Wound-legal definition and types? electrical injuries; thermal injuries; mechanical asphyxia, hanging, strangulation; drowning; suffocation.

U. Sudden Infant Death Syndrone
Definitin; types (cot death, crib death).

V. Maltreatment of Children
Evidence of neglect, physical abuse, sexual abuse, child battering; infanticide.

W. Poisoning
Definition, types-carbon monoxide and other gases, inorganic and organic poisons, venom.

V CHEMISTRY

A. Introductory General Chemistry
Definition; divisions of chemistry; metric system; matter; types of matter based upon composition; energy; changes in matter; the atom; the ion; the molecule; valence; reactions; physical states of matter; solutions; selected elements—nonmetals; selected compounds—water; ionization, air components.

B. Organic Chemistry
Definition; carbon properties; formulas in organic chemistry; classes of organic compounds—aliphatic or open chain (hydrocarbons, organic halides, alcohols, aldehydes, ketones, acids, esters, ethers, amines); ring or closed chain compounds (carbocyclic compounds).

C. Biochemistry, Physiological Chemistry Carbohydrates (hexoses only); fats and oils; proteins; enzymes.

D. Embalming Chemistry
Actions of preservative chemicals; preservation by formaldehyde; embalming fluids- components and functions of arterial and cavity fluids, accessory fluids; factors influencing stability of fluids.

E. Toxicology
Definition of toxicology, toxin, poison, antidote; hazardous character of chemicals used in embalming or present around the mortuary, examples.

VI ANATOMY

A. Introduction and Orientation
Objectives of anatomy course; definitions of anatomy, physiology, gross anatomy, histology, cytology, systemic anatomy, regional anatomy, pathological anatomy, topographical anatomy; anatomical position; terms of reference used in descriptive anatomy-positions, planes and sections, plan of human structures; organization of the human body; definition and names of major organs in each system; definition and types of tissue; definition of cell and its components.

B. Topographical Anatomy
Linear guide, anatomical guide, anatomical limits; abdominal regions; general topographical points on the human body; regional anatomy.

C. Osteology
Introduction and orientation-definition, functions, organs (206 bones exclusive of sutural and sesamoid), divisions of skeleton, organization of bone, bony landmarks, skeleton-all bones and appropriate points, processes, sinuses, etc. of the skull, ear ossicles, hyoid, vertebral column, sternum, ribs, upers appendages, lower appendages; syndesmology definition, fontanels, ligaments, classification and examples of joint or articulations.

D. Digestive System
Location, divisions or parts, and functions of all organs and accesory organs.

E. Excretory System
Structure and function of kidneys; location and function of urinary tract.

F. Reproductive System
Male-definition of scrotum; location, structure, function of epididymis, ductus deferens, seminal vesicles, ejaculator ducts, penis, prostrate gland. Female-location, structure, function of ovaries and uterine tubes; location, regions, wall, function of uterus; location and function of vagina, external genital organs, breast; definition of menstruation.

G. Respiratory System
Definition of respiration, external and internal; location, structure, function of the respiratory organs; associated structures.

H. Circulatory System
All parts and function of lymph vascular system, structure of lymph vessel lymph and its relation to tissue fluid; all parts and function of blood vascular system, structure of blood vessels;arterial and venous systems; general characteristics, volume, composition, clotting, grouping, function of blood.

I. Endocrine System
Classification of types of glands, location of endocrines, hormone definition.

J. Nervous System
Divisons; brain (parts, ventricles, meninges, cerebrospinal fluid spaces); spinal cord; special senses.

K. Muscular System
Organs of muscular system; definitions of muscle actions; names and general locations of muscles of the head, neck and trunk.

FUNERAL SERVICE ARTS

I. SOCIOLOGY OF FUNERAL SERVICE

A. Orientation
Definition of sociology, related terms-funeral, memorial service, funeral rite; its application and purpose in funeral service-social, cultural (definitions of "culture", related terms-enculturation, customs, mores,taboos, folkways, laws, rules, religion, rite, ritual, ceremony), subcultural (definitions of "subculture", related terms-eographic, religious), ethnic (ethnically ethnocentrism vs. cultural relativism), cultural univ-ersals (definition).

B. Customs and American Funeral Rites
The family, related terms—patriarchal, matriarchal, egalitarian, joint, nuclear, modified extended family system; impact of death of a member on each type of family. Changes from joint to nuclear family Industrialization, urbanization, bureaucratization); death in institutions.

C. Changes in American Funeral Rites
Socio-economic change in the last half century has produced significant changes in funeralization; establishment of funeral home; decrease in direct involvement by the family and friends in preparing the dead for burial; increased responsibility of funeral director-need for increased knowledge in social sciences, counseling ability; funeral cost no longer casket price alone; increase in multi-family home, corporate establishments and its effect; influence of organized religions, related terms-traditional funeral rites, non-traditional funeral rites (humanistic, adaptive), primitive funeral rites, immediate disposition.

II PSYCHOLOGY AND COUNSELING

A. Psychology in Funeral Service
Psychological applications: purposes of funeral rites for survivor and those affected by the death; values in funeralization, human and cultural psychological needs of the bereaved, grief syndrome, manner and cause of death of the deceased and its affect on the bereaved.

B. Funeral Service Counseling
Definitions of counseling and Funeral Service Counselor; counseling approaches applicable to funeral service; objectives of counseling; counselor's functions; skills needed in counseling; methods of skill development; arrangement conference; pre-need, at-need, and post-need counseling.

III FUNERAL DIRECTING

A. Initial Contact with the Family (or their representatives) Following Death Proper attitude toward family; identification of person qualified to give permission for release of the deceased from hospital; steps required between initial notification of death and removal of deceased; ascertain attending physician; attempt to set arrangement conference appointment; identify to the family items and information needed at arrangement conference; identify person(s) who qualify to authorize embalming and/or restorative art and/or autopsy.

B. Arrangements Conference
Identification of items included in the Conference; list of items of information needed for obituary classified or editorial, death certificate, Social Security, Veteran's benefits, active armed forces benefits; list appropriate items commonly used to meet funeral needs of those being served; reasons which require discussion involving the family, clergy, and funeral director regarding visitation hours, time of funeral, and order of service; Funeral Service Agreement Form.

C. American Religious Funerals
Basic Knowledge of funeral rites for the following groups:
Protestant; liturgical, non-liturgical, chapel service. special terminology.
Roman Catholic; special terminology and practices.
Orthodox Jewish; special terminology and practices.
Conservative and Reform Jewish; special terinology and practices.
Christian Science, Greek Orthodox, Jesus Christ of Latter-Day Saints (Morman), Religious Society of Friends (Quaker).

D. Fraternal and Military Groups
Basic knowledge of special rites.

E. History of Funeral Directing and Embalming
Basic knowledge.

IV BUSINESS LAW

    A. Law and Its Enforcement
Definition of law, types of law; judicial process, Federal and State Courts.

    B. Contracts
Nature and classes, definition of contract; offer and acceptance; defective agreements; competency of parties; consideration; illegal contracts; forms of contracts; contract assignment; termination of contracts; remedies for Breach of Contract.

    C. Sales
Personal property; formalities of a sale; transfer of title and rist; warranties of seller; bulk sales law.

    D. Commercial Paper
Nature, promissory notes; drafts; checks; liabilities of the parties; essentials of negotiability; negotiation and discharge; holders in due course; defenses.

    E. Agency and Employment
Creation of agency, operation and termination of agency; employer and employee, labor legislation-Federal Wage and Hour Act definition.

    F. Business Organization
Proprietorship; partnerships; corporations.

    G. Property
Definition of property; classification according to movability; methods of acquiring ownership; lost and abandoned property.

    H. Torts
Moral wrongs; tort and breach of contract; tort and crime; basis of tort liability.

V FUNERAL SERVICE LAW

    A. Mortuary Law
Definition, purposes and significance; sources of mortuary law (common law, case law, statutory law, administrative law); civil and criminal law (torts, crimes, actions at law, actions in equity); the dead human body must reflect three main conditions (it must be dead, it must be human, it must not be totally disintegrated) ; property and property rights in a dead human body; obligations o final dispositon; right to control final disposition; disinterment; postmortem examination; torts involving the dead human body, liability for funeral expenses; the funeral establishment.

    B. Probate Law
Wills (requirements revocation, distribution under, testator provisions possible); intestacy (order of distribution, method of distribution); administration of the estate (appointment of personal representative, differences between executor and administrator, priority of claims, insolvent estate, tests for reasonableness of funeral bill, allowable cost items of a funeral) .

VI INTER-AND INTRAPROFESSIONAL RELATIONSHIPS

A. Interprofessional Relationships
Government agencies-Social Security, Veterans Administration benefits, military personnel on active duty death care regulations, burial allowances for civilian employees of armed forces, death of military in United States.

B. Intraprofessional Relationships
Major funeral director associations-National Funeral Directors Association, Order of Golden Rule, National Selected Morticians, Associated Funeral Directors Service, National Funeral Directors and Morticians Association, Jewish Funeral Directors of America, Federated Funeral Directors of America; ethical conduct of funeral service licensee; American Board of Funera Service Education, function and membership; The Conference of Funeral Service Examining Boards, Inc.

VII FUNERAL MERCHANDISE

A. Caskets
Distinguish between casket and coffin, materials used in casket construction-wood, ferrous metals, non-ferrous metals, lastics and fiberglass; component parts of a casket 0 shell, handles, interior, exteriors; style of cap opening-square, round, elliptic, urn; closure methods-sealed caskets; casket sizes.

B. Outer Enclosures
Vaults-purpose, materials commonly used, finishing methods, sealing methods, dimensions, grave liners-purpose, types; transfer containers.

C. Merchandising
Definition, purchasing; service and merchandise proced-ures-pre-selection room counseling, selection room procedures (direct and indirect), post selection room counseling; control-sales frequency chart, inventory.

D. Price Quotation
FTC Rule, content and application.
Unit Pricing-defined, history, advantages, disadvantages; bi-unit pricing-defined, history, advantages, disadvantages; functional pricing-defined, history, advantages, disadvantages, disadvantages, cash advances, define.

VIII ACCOUNTING

A. Accounting Principles
Nature of business accounting; accounting procedure-journalizing transactions, posting to the ledger, trial balance, financial statements; accounting for cash-records of cash receipts and disbursements, petty cash, banking procedures (deposit ticket, checks, endorsements, bank statement, reconciling bank statement, stop payment orders dishonored checks); accounting for personal service enterprise; accounting for merchandise, accounting for notes and interest, accrual accounting applied to retail busness-principles and procedures, application; the periodic summary; adjusting and closing accounts at end of accounting period.

B. Financial Analysis
Income statement analysis-comparative forms, percentage method; balance sheet analysis—comparative forms, ratios, inventory turnover, accounts receivable ratio; comparison of income statement information with balance sheet information—return on capital investment, investment turnover, sources of comparison—history of firm, area pricing, statistics from funeral service organizations or associations, other professional firms, statistics from managerial or governmental publications.

Basic Fundamentals of Anatomy and Physiology

CONTENTS

SECTION	Page
A. Body Structure and Physiology	1
B. The Skeletal System	1
C. The Muscular System	13
D. The Nervous System	18
E. The Circulatory System	23
F. The Respiratory System	25
G. The Digestive System	31
H. The Endocrine System	35
I. The Urinary System	37
J. The Reproductive System	37
K. The Integumentary System	41
L. The Organs as They Occupy the Thoracic and Abdominal Cavities	43

Basic Fundamentals of Anatomy and Physiology

SECTION A—BODY STRUCTURE AND PHYSIOLOGY

1. Introduction. Operating room personnel must know how organs and systems normally work if they are to understand what is happening during surgical procedures. It is well to think in terms of the functions and of the physiology of the body parts while trying to understand anatomy. Avoid a tendency to think in terms of the anatomical structure on which an operation is being performed. The physiological considerations are also helpful in planning operative setups.

2. Planes, Surfaces, Quadrants, and Positions. The importance of planes, surfaces, quadrants, and positions, as illustrated in figures 1 through 4, cannot be overemphasized. The ability to identify the different positions, as well as place patients in them, is an everyday requirement. Planes are necessary in understanding body motion and direction. Figures 2 and 3 show how body areas are used to describe operative sites. The surgeon often refers to the surface area or the abdominal quadrant through which the incision is made.

3. Body Cavities. The body is divided into two main cavities which are readily identified by looking at a midsagittal section of the body, as illustrated in figure 3-5. These are:

a. *The ventral cavity* which encompasses the thoracic cavity, diaphragm, and peritoneal cavity.

b. *The dorsal cavity* which encompasses the cranial and spinal cavities.

4. Cells. A cell is the structural unit of organic life. Each cell contains a nucleus, cytoplasm, and a cell wall, as illustrated in figure 6. Cells differ in size, shape, chemical composition, and special function within the body. They possess the ability to absorb food and secrete waste, grow in size, reproduce, be irritated, and move.

5. Tissue. When a great number of similar cells are combined, they become visible to the naked eye and in this form are referred to as tissue. Figure 7 shows examples of several types of cells and the manner in which they arrange themselves into the *four main kinds of tissue: epithelial, connective, muscle,* and *nerve tissue.* Table 1 shows some of the body areas in which the different types of tissue are located and the function in each location.

6. Membranes. Membranes are the coverings and linings of the body organs and surfaces. The membranes are actually composed of thin sheets of tissue (usually epithelial and connective), which have been so compounded that they are able to *provide protection, absorb moisture, secrete body fluids, regulate heat, eliminate waste, and receive sensory stimulation.* These functions are performed through *cutaneous, synovial, serous,* or *mucous membranes.*

SECTION B—THE SKELETAL SYSTEM

7. Function of the Skeletal System. The skeletal system is the bony framework of the body. It supports the body in an upright position, protects vital organs, and affords attachment for tendons, muscles, and ligaments. It provides the leverage which, by muscular contraction, permits body movements. Blood cells (red blood cells) are formed in the marrow of bones, and bones act as reservoirs for calcium and other minerals.

8. Bones. Bones consist of a hard, outer shell called compact bone and a spongy, porous center called cancellous bone. The center of long bones is called the medullary canal and contains bone marrow. This is the manufacturing center for red blood cells. At the end of long bones is a smooth, glossy tissue which forms the joint surfaces. The surfaces articulate with, fit into, or move in contact with, similar surfaces of other bones. Bone is covered with a thin membrane called periosteum, which is important in the nourishment of bones. It contains nerves and blood vessels and is essential for bone growth. The periosteum, as well as other parts of the bone, are shown in figure 8.

a. If a bone is closely examined, one can see many projections and depressions. The terms listed below are commonly used to describe these areas:

(1) Condyle—a rounded process at the articular (joint) end of a bone.

(2) Crest—a prominent ridge.

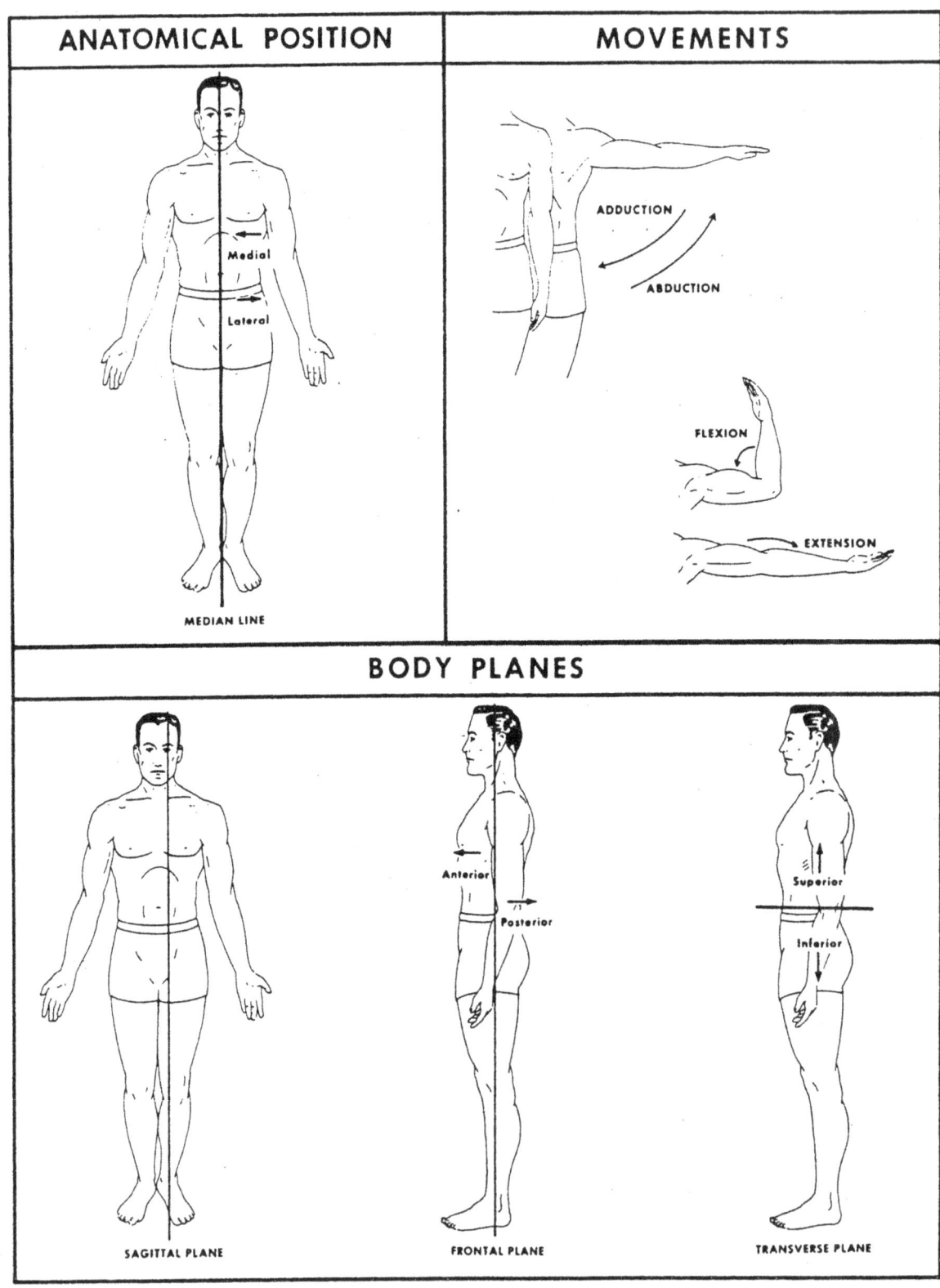

Figure 1. Body Planes and Movements.

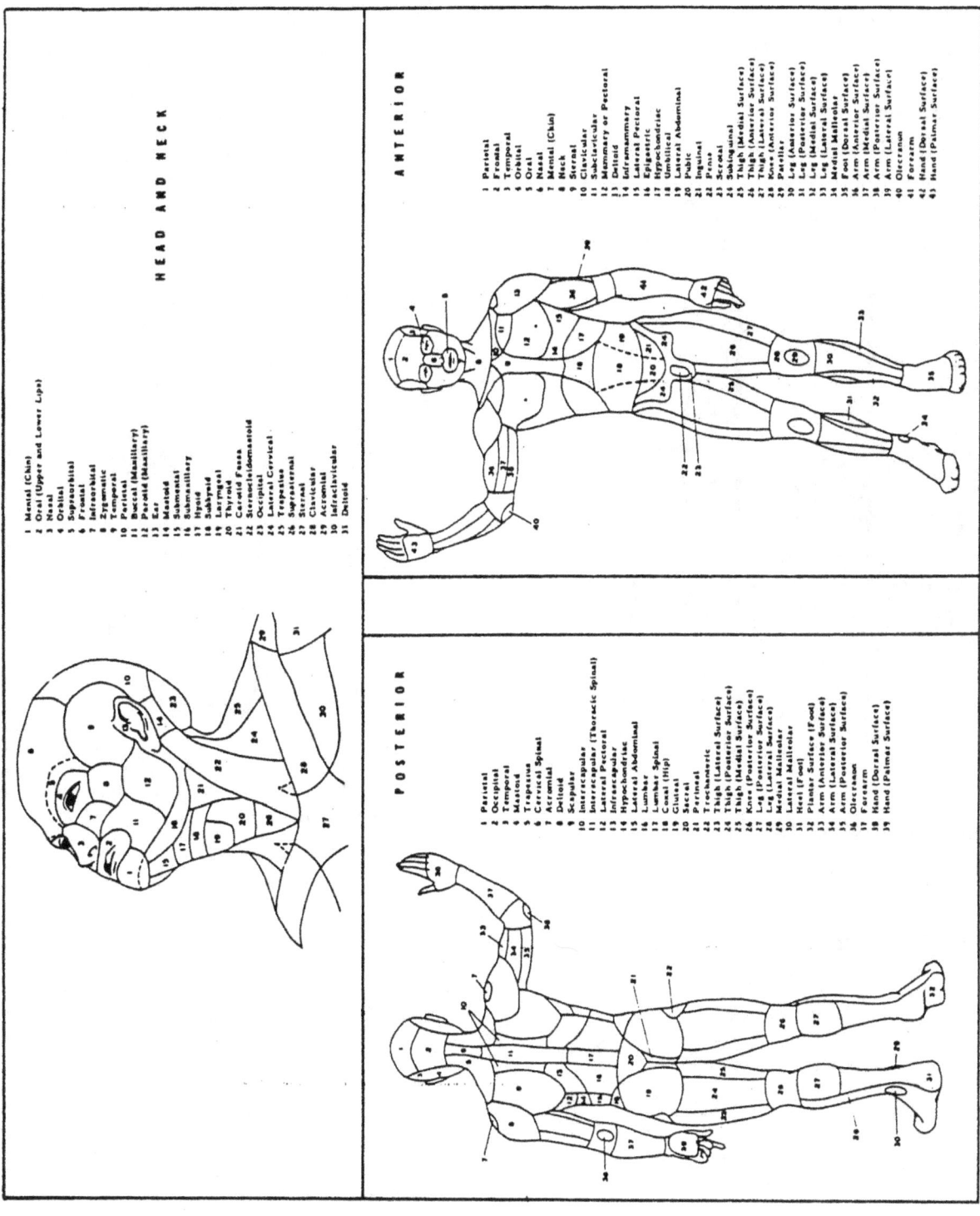

Figure 2. Body Surfaces.

1. Epigastric
2. Upper right quadrant
3. Upper left quadrant
4. Right lateral or lumbar
5. Umbilical
6. Left lateral or lumbar
7. Lower right quadrant (right inguinal)
8. Pubic (hypogastric)
9. Lower left quadrant (left inguinal)

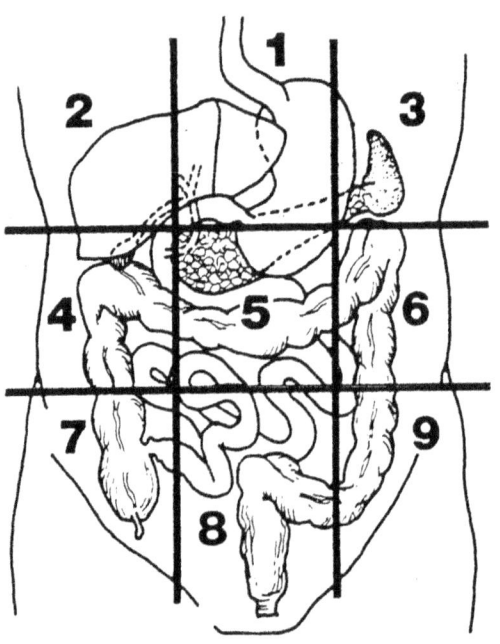

Figure - 3. Anatomic Regions of the Abdomen.

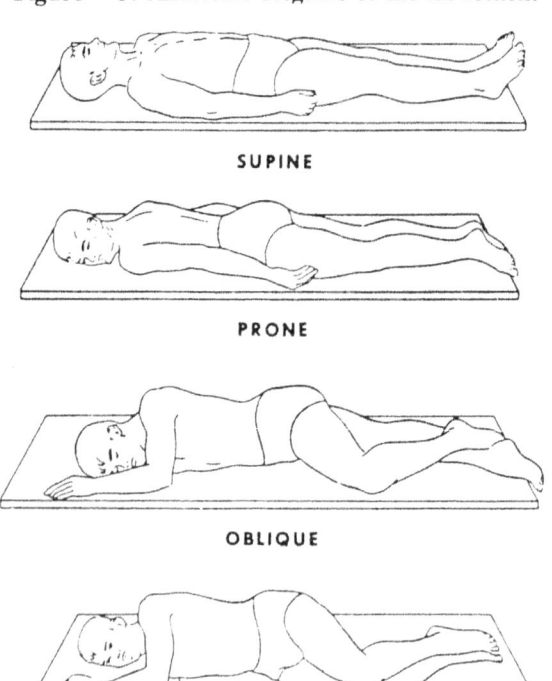

Figure 4. Body Positions.

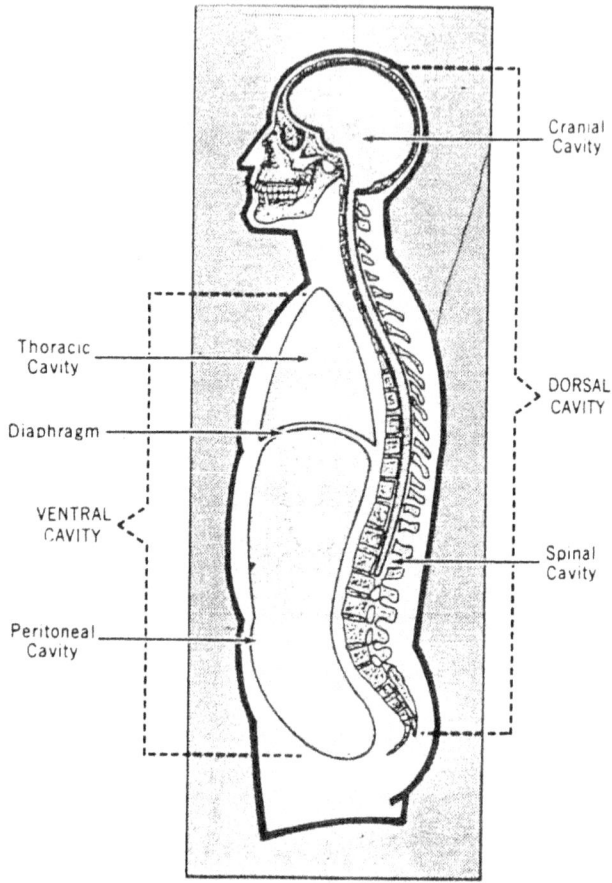

Figure 5. Diagram of Body Cavities as Seen in Midsagittal Section.

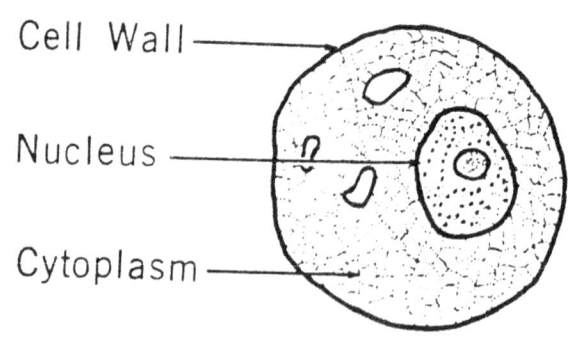

Figure 6. Structure of a Cell.

TYPES OF TISSUES

EPITHELIAL

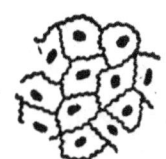
Squamous

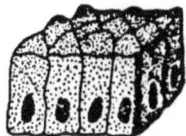
Columnar

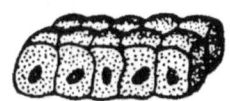
Cuboidal

CONNECTIVE

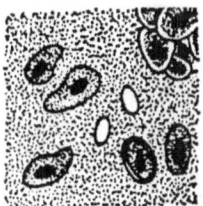
Cartilage

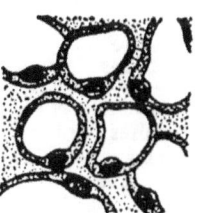
Lymphatic

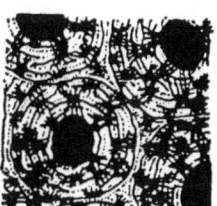
Bone

MUSCLE

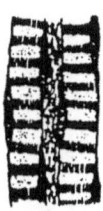
Voluntary

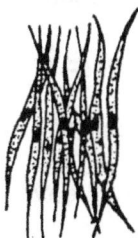
Involuntary

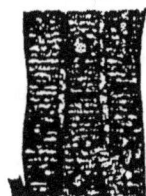
Cardiac

NERVE

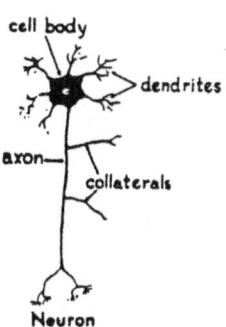
Neuron

Figure 7. Body Cells and Tissues.

Table 1. Body Tissue.

BODY TISSUE

Type of Tissue	Where Located	Purpose
1. Epithelial	Skin Lining of passageways and cavities	Protection Absorption Secretion
2. Connective	Between organs and tissue Walls of vessels Skeleton Blood	Support Elasticity Insulation Protection Transportation of nutrients and waste
3. Muscle	Attached to bones Walls of organs Heart wall	Movement Support, elasticity Heart contractions
4. Nerve	Nerves Brain Spinal cord	Receive stimuli Conduct impulses Effect responses

(3) Diaphysis—the shaft or body of a long bone.

(4) Epiphysis—the end of a long bone.

(5) Fontanelle—an unossified, membranous area usually found in the infant cranium.

(6) Foramen—a hole in a bone for passage of vessels or nerves.

(7) Head—the enlarged portion at the end of a bone.

(8) Process—a general term for any bony prominence.

(9) Sinus—a cavity in a bone.

(10) Spine or spinous process—a slender projection.

b. Bones are classified according to their location and shape. Examples of bones classified according to their shape are as follows:

(1) Long Bones—femur and humerus.

(2) Short Bones—wrists and ankles.

(3) Flat Bones—skull, shoulder, and sternum.

(4) Irregular Bones—mandible and vertebrae.

9. The Skull. The skull is the framework enclosing the brain. It is divided into two parts—the cranium and the face. It is made-up of 22 bones, 8 forming the cranium and 14 forming the face. The cranial bones support and protect the brain and are very firmly united to each other. The junctions of these bones along their edges are called sutures. Cranial bones include one frontal, one occipital, one sphenoid, one ethmoid, two parietal, and two temporal. These bones, along with the facial bones, are shown in figures 9 and 3-10.

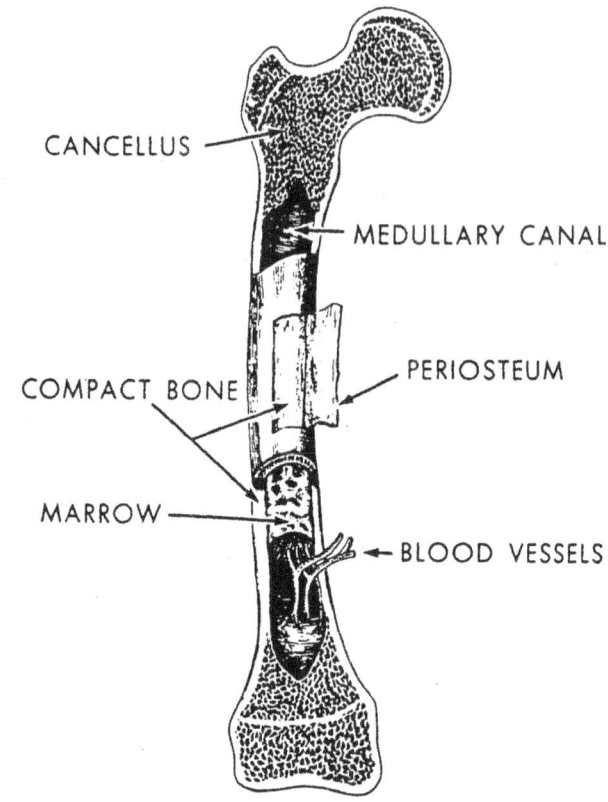

Figure 8. A Long Bone.

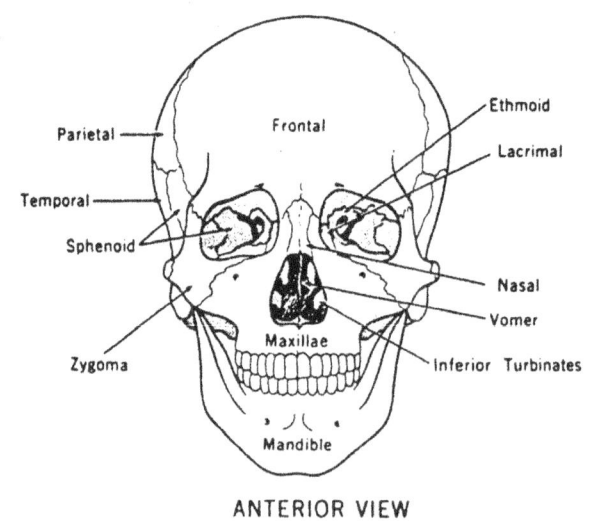

Figure 9. Anterior View of the Skull.

10. The Vertebral Column. The vertebral column consists of 24 movable or true vertebrae, the sacrum, and the coccyx. It is divided into five regions: cervical (neck), thoracic (chest), lumbar (lower back), and the sacral and coccygeal (both in the pelvis). The vertebral column (with its different regions) is shown in figure 11.

a. *Functions of the Vertebrae.* The vertebrae are designed to support and provide motion for the body and extremities, and to serve as a bony protection for the spinal cord, from which nerves arise. A typical vertebra consists of an anterior portion or body and a posterior portion or arch. The body of the vertebra provides support not only for the spinal cord but for other organs of the body as well. Many of the main muscles are also attached to the body of the vertebrae. The various surfaces and processes enable the vertebrae to move upon one another.

b. *Intervertebral Disks.* Between the vertebrae are intervertebral disks. They act as shock absorbers for the vertebral column. They contain an elastic, pulpy substance called nucleus pulposus. A rupture of one of these disks, especially those between the fourth and fifth lumbars, and the fifth lumbar and the sacrum, is a fairly common occurrence. It is termed "herniated nucleus pulposus" (HNP).

c. *Lamina.* The lamina is part of the vertebral arch connected to the pedicles of the vertebra. The laminae are identified in figure 11.

11. The Thorax. The thorax is a cone-shaped, bony cage formed by the 12 thoracic vertebrae, the ribs that terminate anteriorly in articulating cartilages, and the sternum. It houses the heart and lungs. The ribs are curved, flat bones that form most of the posterior and anterior structure and all of the lateral structure of the bony thorax. There are 12 ribs on each side of the thorax, extending from the first through the twelfth thoracic vertebrae. Ribs are identified by number and by the side of the body on which they are located. The first seven pairs are considered true ribs because they are attached to the thoracic vertebrae and to the sternum. The remaining five pairs are considered false ribs because they do not articulate directly with the sternum. The ribs from one to seven become progressively larger; after the seventh rib, they become progressively smaller. The sternum, commonly called the breastbone, is long and flat and is located at the midanterior part of the thoracic cage. It protects the heart, lungs, and greater vessels. The sternum consists of three portions: the manubrium, the body, and the xiphoid process. The entire bony thorax is shown in figure 12.

12. The Upper Extremities. Each upper extremity, shown in figure 13, consists of the clavicle, shoulder, arm, forearm, wrist, and hand.

a. *The Clavicle.* The clavicle, or collarbone, forms the anterior part of the shoulder girdle. It lies in a horizontal position just above the first rib. It is attached to the scapula and the sternum. Because of its anterior location, it is often fractured as a result of a fall.

b. *The Scapula.* The scapula (shoulder bone) is a triangular-shaped bone lying in the upper part of the back. It forms the posterior portion of the shoulder girdle and a part of the shoulder joint.

c. *The Humerus.* The humerus is the bone of the upper arm and is classified as a long bone. It articulates with the shoulder girdle to form the shoulder joint and the bones of the forearm to form the elbow joint.

d. *The Forearm.* The bones of the forearm are called the ulna and the radius. From an anatomical position, the radius is on the lateral or thumb side with the ulna on the medial or little finger side. The ulna and radius articulate at their proximal ends with the humerus and at their distal ends with some of the carpal bones.

e. *The Wrist and Hand.* The wrist and hand are made up of 27 separate bones. The wrist contains eight small bones called carpals. The hand consists of 5 metacarpal bones and 14 phalanges. The metacarpal bones are numbered one to five to correspond to the five fingers. The phalanges are the small bones of the fingers and thumb.

13. The Lower Extremities. The bones that make up the lower extremities are the innominate

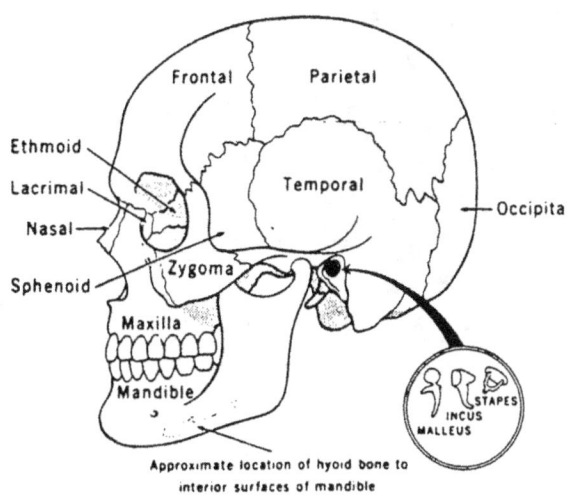

LATERAL VIEW

Figure 10. Lateral View of the Skull.

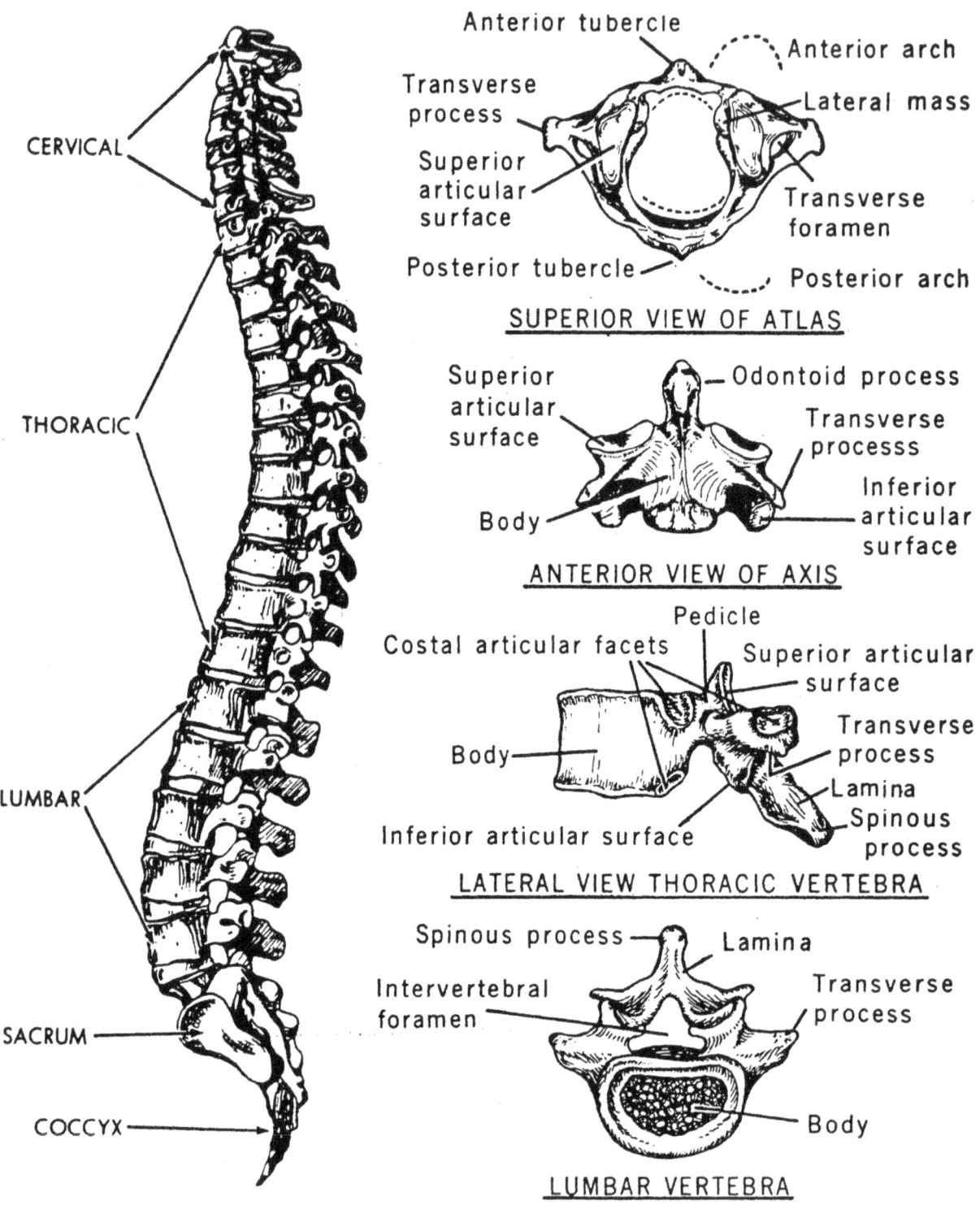

Figure 11. Vertebral Column.

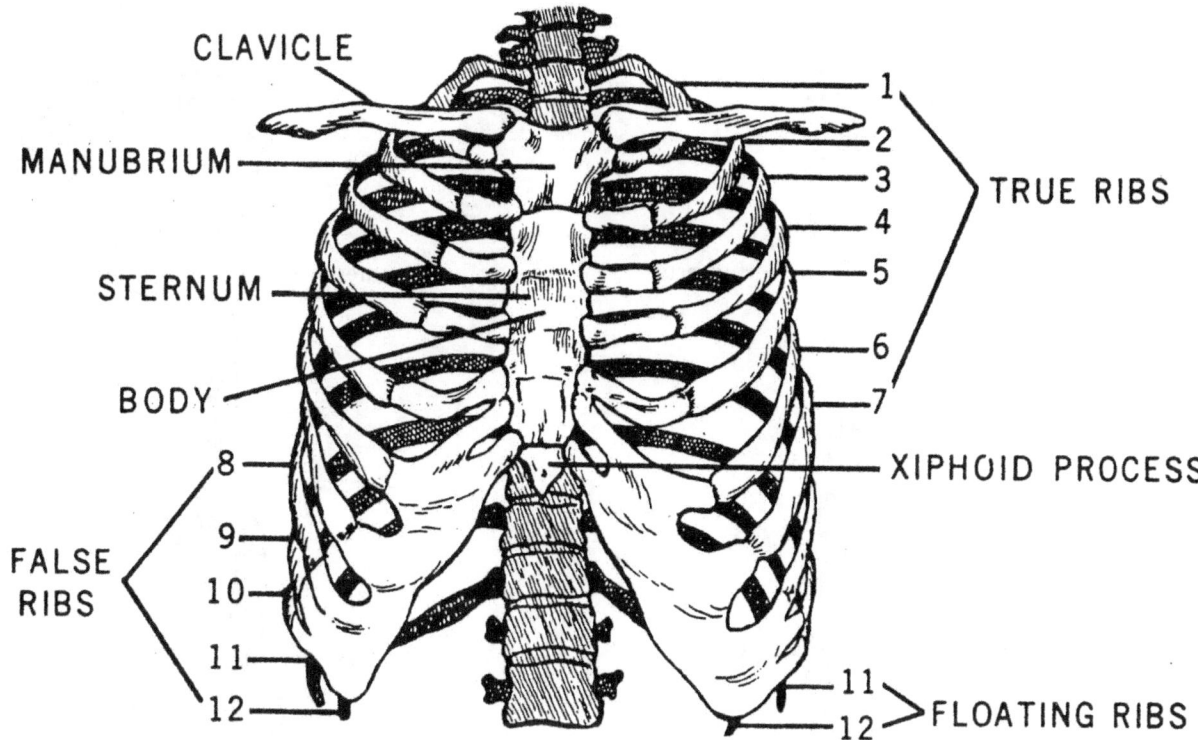

Figure 12. Bony Thorax, Anterior Aspects.

(hipbone), femur, patella, tibia and fibula, tarsals, metatarsals, and the phalanges. Each of these bones is shown in figure 14.

a. *The Pelvic Girdle.* The two hipbones, together with the sacrum and coccyx posteriorly, form the pelvic girdle. This girdle forms a deep basin, which protects the organs of the lower abdomen, the bladder, lower bowel, and reproductive organs.

b. *The Femur.* The femur, or thigh bone, is the longest bone in the body. The proximal end is rounded and has a head that fits into the acetabulum. It also has a neck, the part of the femur most frequently fractured.

c. *The Lower Leg.* The bones of the lower leg are the tibia and fibula. The tibia is the inner and larger bone; it articulates with the femur and the head of the fibula at the top and the talus at the bottom. The fibula is the outer and smaller bone. The fibula is most often fractured, but a fracture of the tibia is generally more serious.

d. *The Ankle and Foot.* The bones of the foot are similar in structure and arrangement to those of the hand. They include the 7 tarsals, 5 metatarsals, and 5 phalanges. The tarsals form the anklebones, and the metatarsals form the sole and instep of the foot. The phalanges form the toes.

14. Joints. The place of union between two or more bones of the skeleton is a joint. Because of the way the bones are attached, the body position can be changed, and hundreds of motions are possible. Figure 15 illustrates range of motion, as used in exercises and orthopedic positions.

a. *Anatomy.* The joints are lined with a membrane that secretes a fluid called synovial fluid. This fluid serves as a lubricant and keeps the joint working smoothly. Cartilage plates cover the ends of the bones and provide a smooth surface for rotation in freely movable joints. When the bones meet to form a joint, they require assistance to stay in place. This is the responsibility of the ligaments. The bursae are sacs filled with a viscid fluid and located between the ends of bones to act as a cushion. They are also found between muscle and bone or between tendons.

b. *Types of Joints.* Joints are of three different types: immovable, slightly movable, and freely movable. Figure 16 illustrates each of these types of joints.

(1) *Immovable.* In immovable joints, the surfaces of the bones are almost in direct contact and are fastened together with a thin layer of intervening fibrous tissue or cartilage. An example of this type of joint is the joining of the bones of the skull.

(2) *Slightly Movable.* In slightly movable joints, the bony surfaces are connected by broad, flattened disks of fibrocartilage or by a fibrous ligament between the bones. Examples of this type of joint

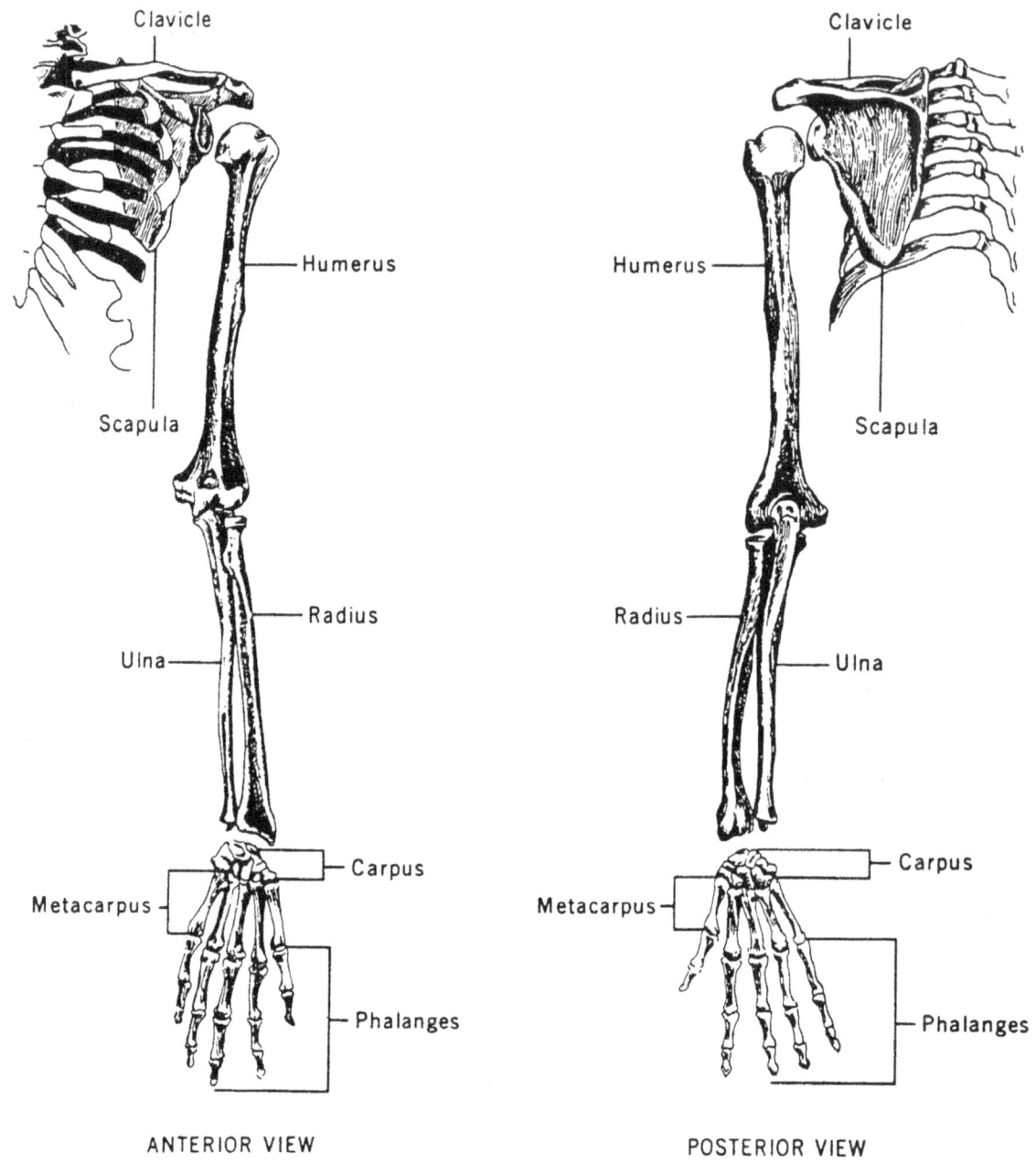

Figure 13. Upper Extremities.

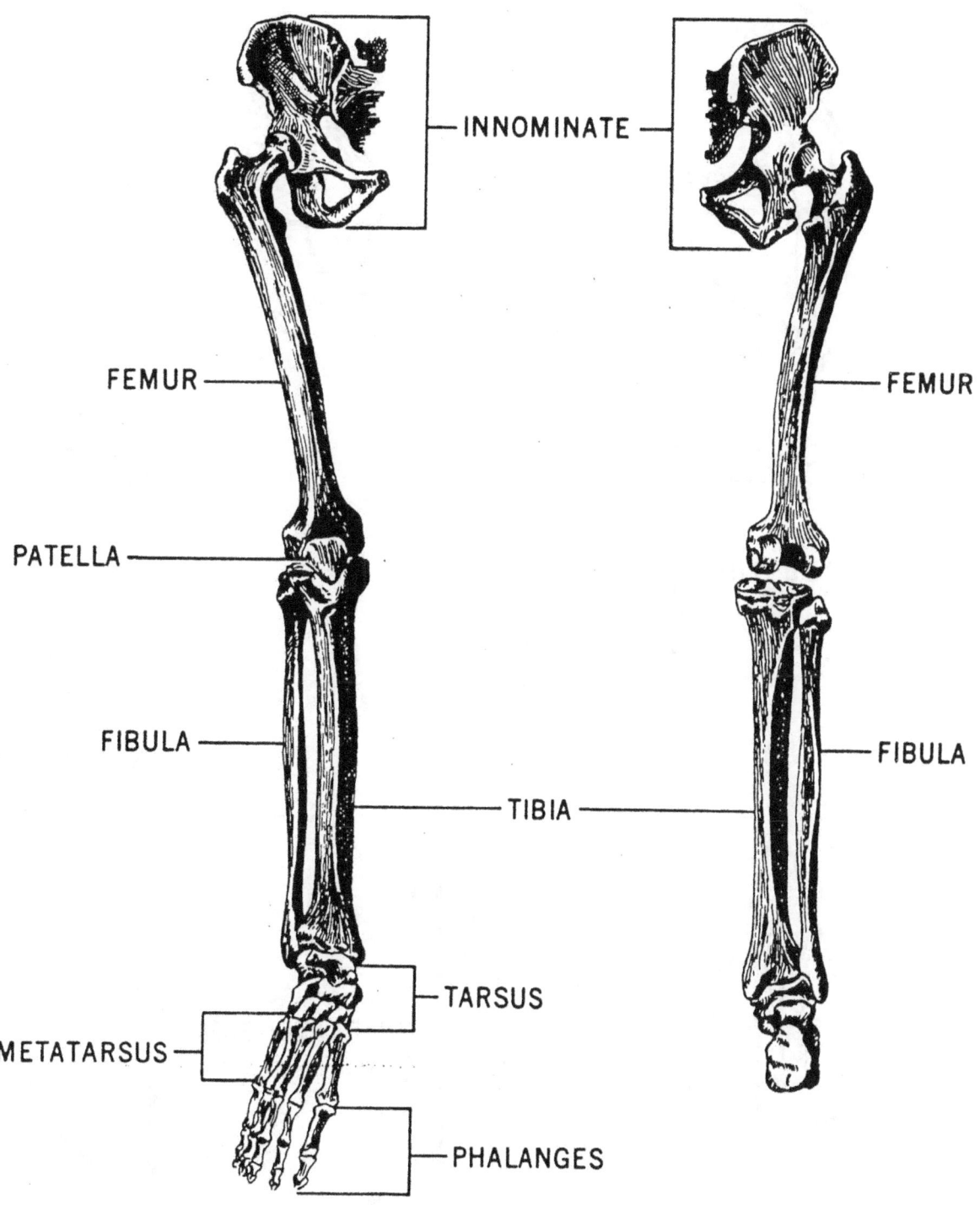

Figure 14. Lower Extremities.

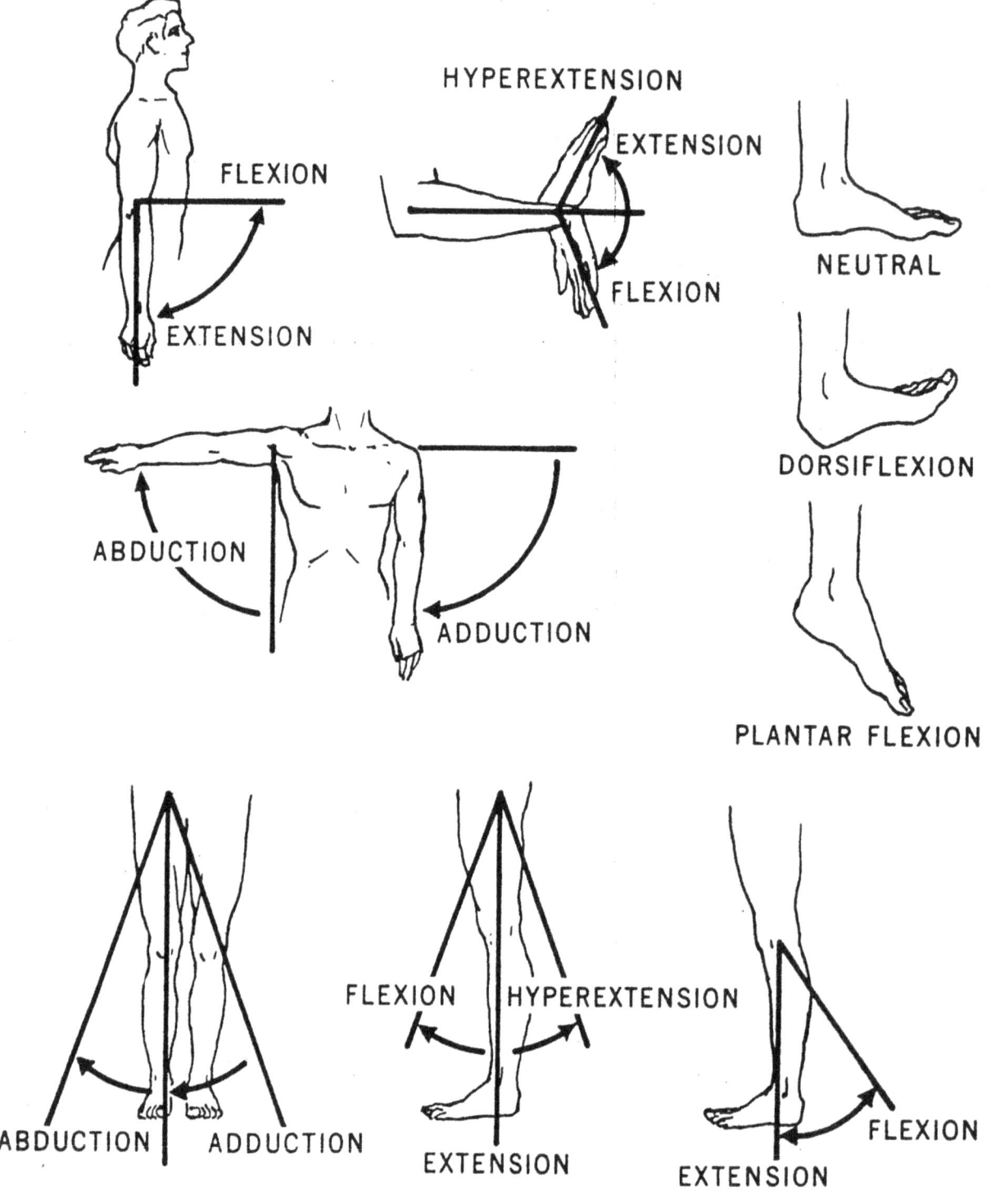

Figure 15. Range of Motion.

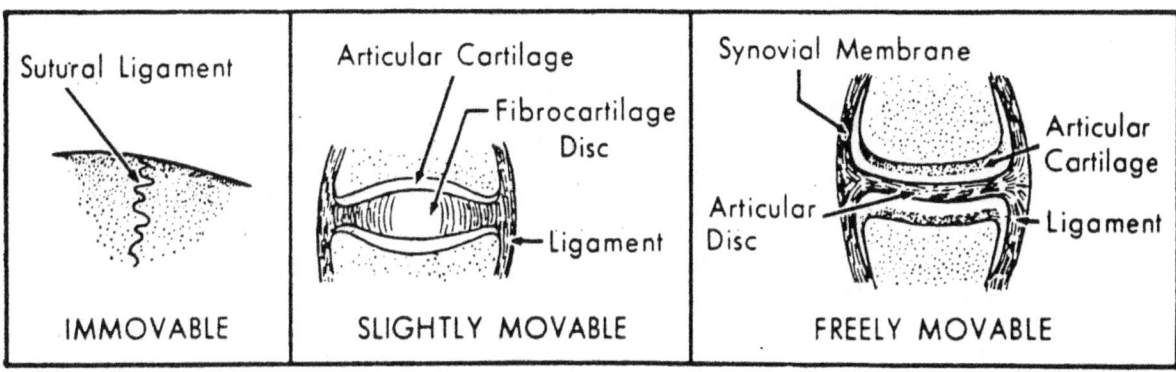

Figure 16. Types of Joints.

are the articulations of the bones of the vertebrae and the symphysis pubis.

(3) *Freely Movable.* Freely movable joints are the most numerous in the body and have a more complex arrangement. The surface of each bone is covered with articular cartilage. The bones are connected by ligaments that pass from one to the other on all sides of the joint, thus forming a capsule. This articular capsule is made up of two layers of tissue. The outer layer is fibrous tissue; the inner layer is the synovial membrane and secretes synovial or lubricating fluid. Some joints are divided completely or incompletely by a disk that is continuous with the articular capsule. Movable joints are classified according to the types of motion permitted by their structures. Some of the main types are:

(a) Hinge joints, such as the elbow and knee.

(b) Ball-and-socket joints, in which the round head of one bone fits into a cuplike cavity of another, such as the shoulder and hip.

(c) Gliding joints, where the surfaces of adjacent bones glide upon each other, such as those of the wrist and ankle.

(d) Pivot (or rotary) joints, where one bone pivots or rotates about another that is stationary, such as the axis about the atlas.

(e) Condyloid joints, in which an oval head of one bone fits into a shallow depression of another, as the carpal bones fit into the finger bones.

15. Overview of the Skeletal System. The skeletal system includes some 206 bones and numerous ligaments and cartilages which make up the joints that attach the bones together. Table 2 lists all of the bones along with their location and body area.

SECTION C—THE MUSCULAR SYSTEM

16. Functions of the Muscular System. The muscular system is important not only because muscular contraction results in movement, locomotion, and maintenance of erect posture, but also because it is involved in such essential bodily functions as pumping the blood around the body and in respiration and digestion.

17. Voluntary and Involuntary Muscles. Muscle is a tissue composed of a number of fibers held together by connective tissue and enclosed in a fibrous sheath called fascia. Muscles are characterized by their ability to contract and, thereby, to move the various parts of the body. All motion of the body, whether conscious or unconscious, is due to action of the muscles. All muscle is normally in a state of partial tension at all times and, therefore, is said to have tone or tonus. The tendency to contract is present throughout life so that if a muscle is cut, the two ends pull apart just as do the cut ends of a stretched rubber band. The muscle tissues of the body vary in shape and structure according to the functions they perform. They are divided into two main groups—voluntary muscles and involuntary muscles.

a. *Voluntary Muscles.* A muscle that is under conscious control is a voluntary muscle. All the muscles attached to the skeleton are of the voluntary type. Groups of muscle bundles held together by fascia make up the individual muscle, each of which is named according to its location, action, or other distinguishing feature. Each skeletal muscle is made up of three main parts—the origin, the belly, and the insertion. The origin is the point where the muscle is anchored, and it usually consists of a short tendon attached to the bone. The belly is the largest part of the body and is made up of many fibers. The insertion is the point on which the action of the muscle is applied, resulting in motion. Here the muscle is attached to a bone by a tendon. Tendons are nonelastic, dense, fibrous tissue. They unite with the periosteum of bones to form secure attachments for the muscles.

b. *Involuntary Muscles.* A muscle whose nerve

Table 2. Skeletal Bones.

SKELETAL BONES

Body Area	Bone	Number in the body	Location
Axial Skeleton (80 bones) 1. Skull (29 bones) a. Cranium (8 bones)	1. Frontal 2. Occipital 3. Sphenoid 4. Ethmoid 5. Parietal 6. Temporal	1 1 1 1 2 2	Forehead Base of skull Across midportion of cranial floor Front of cranial floor Bulging two top portions of skull Lower two sides, anterior and superior to ears.
b. Face (14 bones)	1. Nasal 2. Mandible 3. Vomer 4. Maxilla 5. Zygomatic 6. Lacrimal 7. Inferior turbinates 8. Palatine	2 1 1 2 2 2 2 2	Bridge of nose Lower jaw Lower part of nasal system Upper jaw Cheek bones Lateral to nasal bones Inner surface of nasal side wall Roof of mouth
c. Ear (6 bones)	1. Malleus (hammer) 2. Incus (anvil) 3. Stapes (stirrups)	2 2 2	Hammer-shaped bone in middle ear Anvil-shaped bone in middle ear Stirrup-shaped bone in middle ear
d. Tongue	1. Hyoid	1	In throat, at root of tongue
2. Chest (25 bones)	1. True ribs 2. False ribs 3. Sternum	7 pairs 5 pairs 1	Attached to sternum 3 upper pairs attached to cartilage. 2 lower pairs are floating. Breast bone
3. Spine (26 bones)	1. Cervical vertebrae 2. Thoracic vertebrae 3. Lumbar vertebrae 4. Sacrum 5. Coccyx	7 12 5 1 1	First 7 vertebrae (neck) Next 12 vertebrae (chest area) Next 5 vertebrae (small of back) Lower end of spine (contains 5 fused bones) Remains of a tail (contains 4 fused bones)
Appendicular Skeleton (126 bones) 1. Upper Extremities (64 bones)	1. Clavicle 2. Scapula 3. Humerus 4. Radius 5. Ulna 6. Carpals 7. Metacarpals 8. Phalanges	2 2 2 2 2 16 10 28	Collar bone Shoulder blade Upper arm Forearm, thumb side Forearm, little finger side Wrist bones Palm of hands Fingers and thumbs
2. Lower Extremities (62 bones)	1. Innominate bone 2. Femur 3. Patella 4. Tibia 5. Fibula 6. Tarsal 7. Metatarsal 8. Phalanges	2 2 2 2 2 14 10 28	Hip or pelvis Thigh Knee cap Shin Calf side of lower leg Ankle Foot Toes

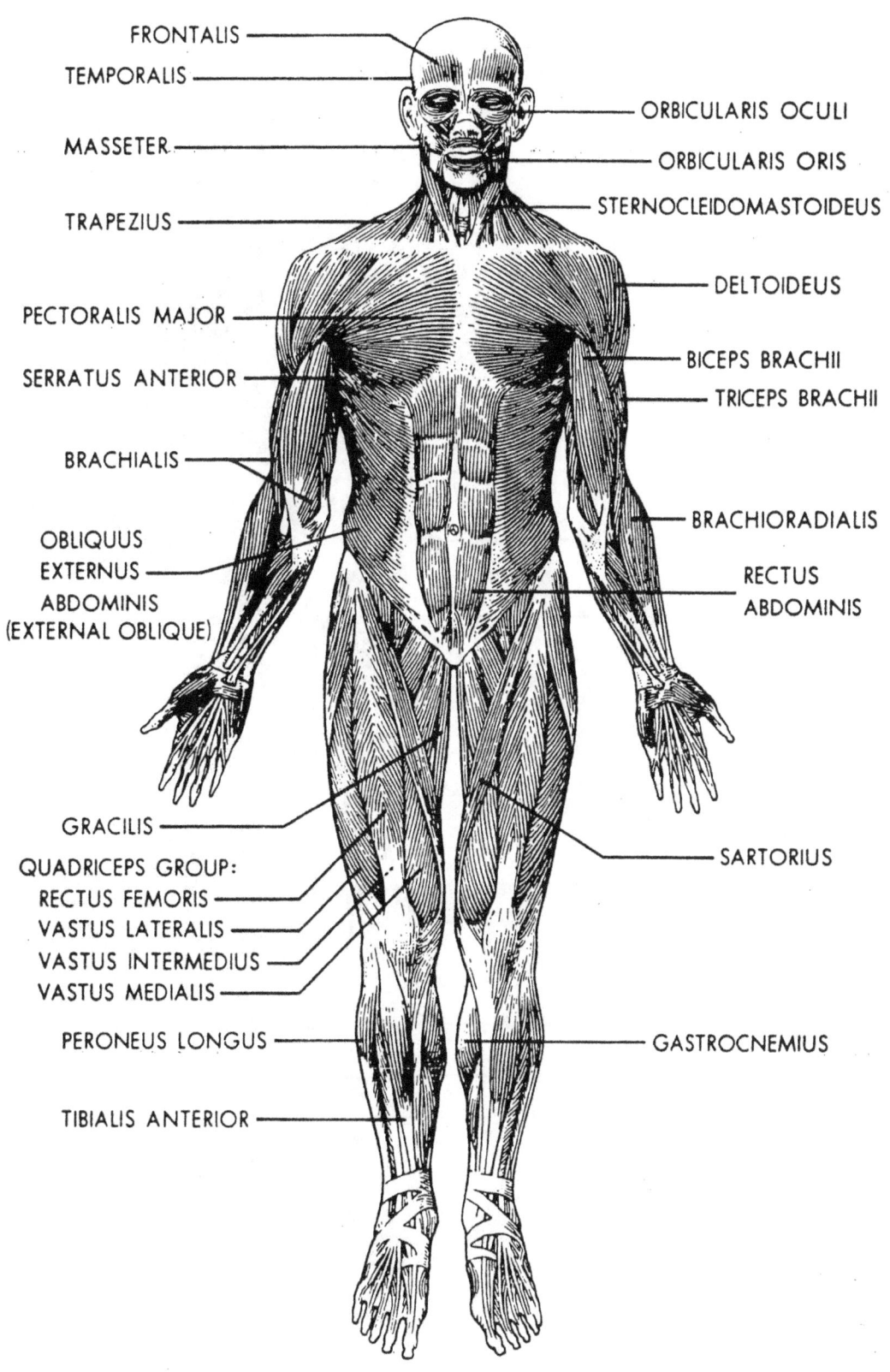

Figure 17. Anterior Superficial Muscles.

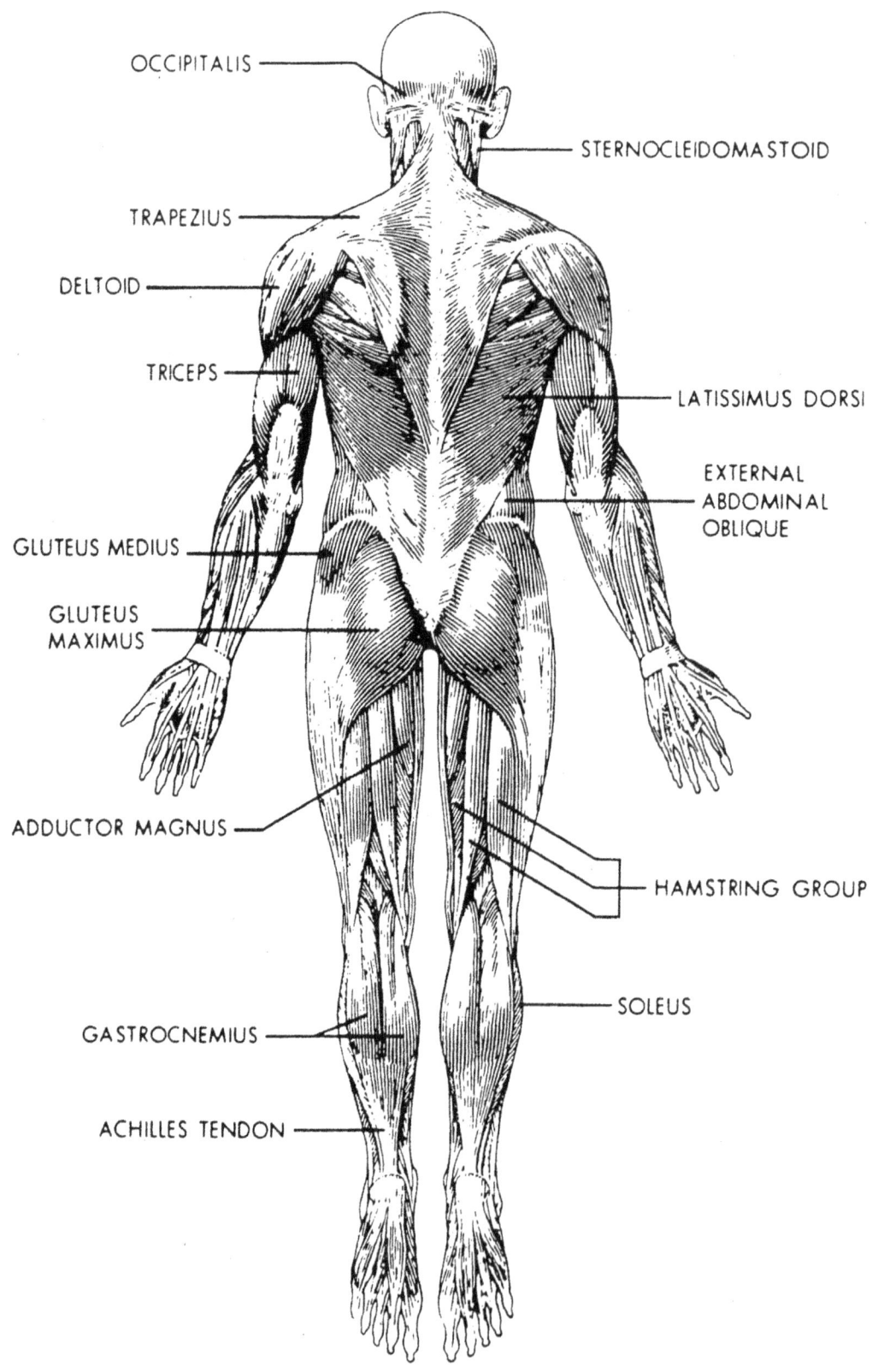

Figure 18. Posterior Superficial Muscles.

supply comes from the autonomic nervous system (the part of our nervous system over which we have no direct control) is an involuntary muscle. These muscles are found in the walls of the blood vessels, in the intestinal tract, and in the glands. Their action is well illustrated in the intestinal tract, where they push food along by rhythmic contractions (peristalsis). A special kind of involuntary muscle is the cardiac muscle. Its structure is quite different from that of any other muscle.

18. Muscles of the Upper and Lower Extremities. The major muscles and muscle groups are illustrated in figures 17 and 18.

a. *Upper Extremities.* The major muscles of the upper extremities consist of the deltoid, the biceps brachii, and the triceps brachii. The first of these, the deltoid, fits as a "cap" over the shoulder and occupies the superolateral portion of the shoulder prominence. It is widely used for injections. The biceps brachii is a large spindle-shaped muscle forming the major portion of the bulge on the anterior surface of the upper arm. The triceps brachii occupies the posterior surface of the arm.

b. *Lower Extremities.* The lower extremities have several major muscles: the gluteus maximus, the quadriceps, the hamstrings, and the gastrocnemius. The first of these, the gluteus maximus, is the large, fleshy muscle forming the prominence of the buttocks. The quadriceps are a four-headed group of muscles forming the anterior portion of the thigh. The hamstrings are three muscles located on the posterior thigh. The gastrocnemius is the large, superficial muscle forming the major portion of the calf of the leg. It is inserted into the heel bone by the Achilles tendon, the largest tendon in the body.

19. The Abdominal Muscles. There are several different abdominal muscles forming broad, thin layers that support the internal organs. These muscles also assist in breathing, in flexing the thorax on the pelvis, and in flexing and rotating the spine.

20. The Back Muscles. The muscles of the back are large and broad. They are attached to the vertebrae and keep the trunk in an erect position, permitting it to bend and turn. These movements occur mainly in the cervical lumbar regions. Some of the major muscle groups, as well as their location and function, are explained in table 3.

Table 3. Location and Purpose of Major Muscle Groups.

Location	Muscle	Purpose
Head	Occipito frontalis Orbicularis oculi Orbicularis oris Masseter	Raises eyebrows Closes eye Closes lips Closes jaw
Neck	Sternocleidomastoid	Flexes head
Shoulder	Deltoid Trapezius	Abducts upper arm Raises shoulder; extends head
Chest	Pectoralis major	Flexes and adducts anteriorly the upper arm
Abdomen	External abdominal oblique Rectus abdominus Inguinal ligament	Compresses abdomen; flexes trunk Compresses abdomen; flexes trunk Insertion area for external oblique
Back	Latissimus dorsi	Extends upper arm and adducts it posteriorly
Arm	Biceps brachii Triceps brachii Flexors Extensors	Flexes lower arm Extends lower arm Flexes hand Extends hand
Thigh	Gluteus Maximus Adductor group Sartorius Quadriceps femoris Hamstring group	Extends and abducts thigh Adducts and flexes thigh Adducts, flexes and "crosses" lower leg Extends leg; flexes thigh Flexes lower leg
Lower Leg	Gastrocnemius (Achilles tendon) Extensors Soleus	Flexes leg; extends foot Extends toes Extends foot

21. **Muscle Tone.** Muscles are never completely relaxed; they are always in a state of partial contraction. This state is referred to as *muscle tone*, and it involves a complicated chemical process by which glucose is broken down into lactic acid and energy. This process is more active when the muscle is being consciously contracted, extended, or irritated. Even though muscle tone is advantageous for normal body functions, it can become a problem to the surgeons who would, for example, like to have the abdominal muscles relaxed when they explore a peritoneal cavity. The elasticity which allows flexion of the fingers can also cause a severed tendon to retract deep into surrounding tissue, thus necessitating a probing search on the part of a surgeon who is trying to repair the injury. In the case of needed abdominal relaxation, it may sometimes be necessary to inject muscle-relaxing drugs before deep abdominal surgery can be performed. Figure 19 illustrates the number of muscle layers the surgeon must contend with in his approach to the abdominal cavity.

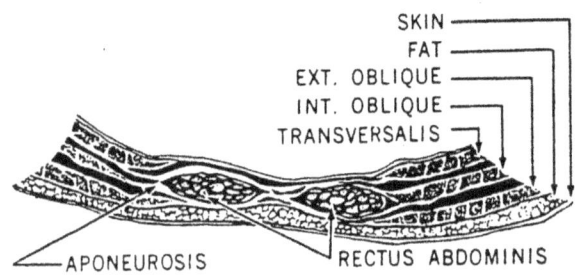

Figure 19. Cross Section of Abdominal Muscle Layers.

SECTION D—THE NERVOUS SYSTEM

22. **Function of the Nervous System.** The nervous system is the means by which the human body is integrated and enabled to function as a whole. The nervous system is the stimulus-response mechanism that coordinates and regulates all body activity. It is responsible for all the processes that make up the adjustment to both internal and external environment. It is the most highly organized system in the body. The nervous system may be considered as an intricate communications system that transmits impulses from different parts of the body to the brain, and from the brain to organs and structures that react to impulses.

23. **Divisions of the Nervous System.** The nervous system is both *voluntary* and *involuntary* and is composed of the brain, spinal cord, nerves, and ganglia. It is also divided into a *central nervous system* (CNS) and a *peripheral nervous system* (PNS). The peripheral nervous system also includes the autonomic nervous system, which is self-controlling and is formed from the many nerves that innervate the internal organs, glands, and blood vessels. Table 4 shows the divisions of the CNS and the PNS.

24. **Neurons.** The basic structural unit of the nervous system is the neuron or nerve cell. Each neuron contains a cell body and cell processes called dendrites and axons. Dendrites carry impulses away from the cell body. A typical nerve cell is shown in figure 7.

Table 4. Divisions of the Nervous System.

DIVISIONS OF THE NERVOUS SYSTEM

Central Nervous System (CNS)	*Peripheral Nervous System (Craniospinal Division)*

Brain:
  Cerebrum
  Cerebellum
  Midbrain
  Pons
  Medulla Oblongata
	Cranial Nerves and their Functions:
	  1. Olfactory (smell)
	  2. Optic (vision)
	  3. Oculomotor (eye movement and pupil size)
	  4. Trochlear (eye movement)
	  5. Trifacial (sensations in face and head, chewing)
	  6. Abducens (abduction of eye)
	  7. Facial (facial expressions and taste)
	  8. Auditory (hearing and equilibrium)
	  9. Glossopharyngeal (taste and swallowing)
	  10. Vagus (various sensations and movements in heart, intestines, etc.)
	  11. Spinal accessory (head and shoulder movement)
	  12. Hypoglossal (tongue movements)

Spinal Cord	Spinal Nerves and Areas Innervated:
	  8 cervical (shoulder, neck, head, chest)
	  12 thoracic (shoulder, chest, arm, hand)
	  5 lumbar (back, hip, thigh, genitalia)
	  5 sacral (rectum, buttocks, leg, foot)
	  1 coccygeal (skin in coccyx area)

25. Afferent and Efferent Neurons. There are two types of neurons—*afferent, which is receptive or sensory,* and *efferent, which is effective or motor.* Afferent neurons carry impulses from the periphery (body) toward the spine and brain. Efferent neurons carry impulses from the brain and spine to the periphery. The bodies of afferent neurons are located in ganglia, just outside the spinal cord. *A ganglion is a group or mass of neurons* that serve as a center of nervous impulses.

26. Nerves. A nerve is a cordlike structure that transmits impulses from one part of the body to another. A nerve has many fibers that are closely associated but have independent functions. A nerve may consist of sensory fibers only, motor fibers only, or a combination of both.

27. The Central Nervous System. The central nervous system is composed of the brain and spinal cord and is contained or located inside the cranial cavity and in the vertebral canal. Figure 20 illustrates the environment of the brain and spinal cord in midsagittal section. The brain, shown in figure 21, receives and interprets impulses and sends out responses.

   a. The *cerebrum* (or forebrain) is the largest part of the brain and is divided into right and left halves called hemispheres. Each hemisphere is divided into specialized lobes, named after the cranial bones to which they join. Each of these lobes is a specialized, functional area. The frontal lobe is a motor area; the parietal lobe is a sensory area; the occipital lobe is the center of vision; and the temporal lobe is the center of hearing.

   b. The cerebrum presents a wrinkled appearance, characterized by many ridges and convolutions. The outer layer of the cerebrum, called the cortex, is made up of gray matter containing nerve cells. It governs all conscious functions. The interior of the cerebrum is white and contains bundles of axons and nerve tracts. Its functions include accumulation and storage of knowledge, or memory, and the interpretation of sensations.

   c. The *cerebellum* is the second largest part of the brain and is located in the lower posterior part of the cranial cavity, beneath the cerebrum. Its primary functions are concerned with the coordination of muscular movements and body balance or equilibrium.

   d. The *brain stem* consists of three functional parts: the midbrain, the pons, and the medulla oblongata. The *midbrain* is a small structure containing nuclei for reflex control. The *pons* makes up the middle part of the brain stem and serves as a bridge to connect the brain stem to the cerebellum. It also serves as a place for the exit of cranial nerves and helps to regulate respiration. The *medulla oblongata* is the part of the brain that connects with the spinal cord. It is the location of such vital control centers as respiration, heartbeat, and blood pressure. In addition, many reflex actions such as sneezing, coughing, and peristaltic movement are also controlled by the medulla.

   e. The *spinal cord* is the main nerve trunk for the body. It is like a large telephone cable, able to carry hundreds of messages at the same time. It is located inside the vertebral column, extending from the brain to the lower region of the back. The spinal cord is the means by which impulses from the brain reach the periphery of the body, and also the way by which impulses from the periphery reach the brain. The spinal cord contains 31 pairs of spinal nerves, with both sensory and motor fibers, that lead from the cord to all parts of the body.

   f. The brain and spinal cord are covered with three layers of special membranes called *meninges*. They serve as protective covering for brain and spinal cord. The space between the middle and inner layers contains cerebrospinal fluid, a clear, watery solution similar to blood plasma. It circulates over the entire surface of the brain and spinal cord and provides a protective cushion as well as a source of nourishment for these structures. The cerebrospinal fluid is continuously being formed by a plexus (network or mass) of blood vessels in the brain, and as it is formed, a like amount is continuously reabsorbed.

28. The Peripheral Nervous System. The peripheral nervous system is made up of 12 pairs of cranial nerves and 31 pairs of spinal nerves stemming from the brain and spinal cord, respectively. These nerves carry both voluntary and involuntary impulses. The cranial nerves are sensory, motor, or mixed.

29. The Autonomic Nervous System. The autonomic nervous system, as shown in figure 22, belongs to the peripheral nervous system and is functional rather than organic. It is formed from the many nerves that innervate the internal organs, glands, and blood vessels. Its action, as the name implies, is automatic. The autonomic nervous system enables the body to maintain an internal environment suitable for all vital body processes. It is further divided into a *sympathetic* and a *parasympathetic* system. These two systems act in opposition to each other. For example, the sympathetic system stimulates nerves which cause acceleration of the heartbeat and a rise in blood pressure. The parasympathetic system acts to slow the heart and lower the blood pressure. By acting in opposition, the two opposing functions tend to keep the body in delicate balance.

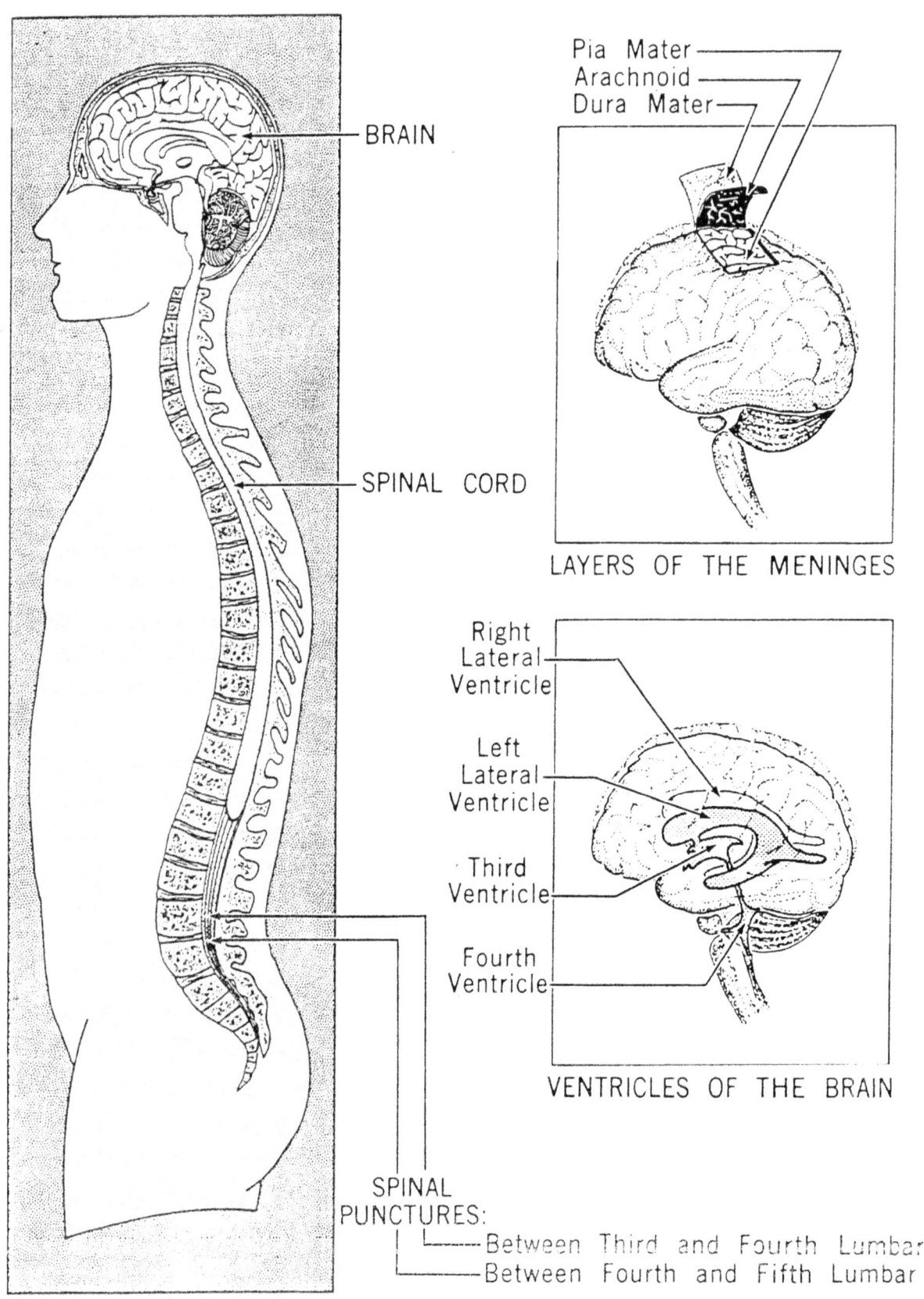

Figure 20. Environment of the Brain and Spinal Cord in Midsagittal Section.

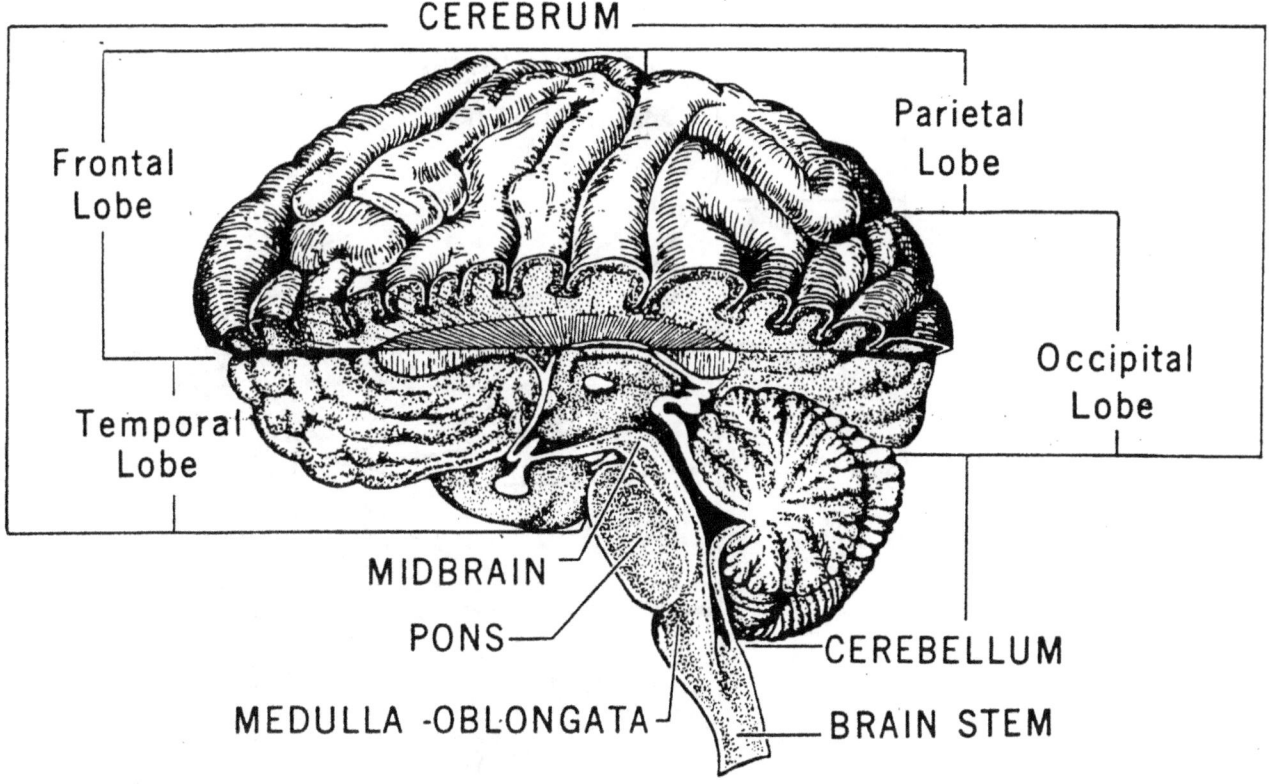

Figure 21. The Brain.

30. The Major Nerve Branches. The major nerve branches are illustrated in figure 23. Each of these branches continues to diverge into numerous fine threads which carry on a communication process throughout the body. It is these fine nerves that conduct local anesthetic agents into the tissues surrounding small operative areas.

31. Sensory Neurons. Sensory neurons carry the impulses into the posterior portion of the cord. They may synapse (connect) with motor neurons at this level, or the cord may act as a cable and transmit the information to the brain for interpretation. Then the responsive impulse is passed down through the anterior portion of the cord, and motor neurons deliver it to the muscle or organ that will react.

  a. Sensations which originate in the skin include heat, cold, pain, touch, and pressure. The receptors for each of these are not evenly distributed throughout the body, and for this reason sensitivity to the different stimuli may vary from one part of the body to another.

  b. The *eye* is a highly specialized sense organ. It is contained in a cone-shaped, bony cavity called the *orbit*. When reflected light rays enter through the *cornea*, shown in figure 24, they are quickly controlled by the shutter action of the *iris* which allows different sizes of *lens* openings. The *ciliary muscle* adjusts the shape of the lens so that light rays are focused to the rear of the eye on the *retina*. From here, the *optic nerve* sends the impression to the brain, and an interpretation is made. Work in the area of the eye must always be concerned with the delicate nature of eye tissue, and with the measures which will protect the patient from pain or injury.

  c. *Hearing* also involves an interpretation by the central nervous system. Sound waves are transferred through the three portions of the ear as illustrated in figure 25. The *outer ear* picks up these sound waves and passes them along a canal or *auditory meatus* until they strike the *tympanic membrane* (ear drum). The vibration produced at this point is transmitted through the middle ear by three small bones, which are shaped like a *hammer* (malleus), an *anvil* (incus), and a *stirrup* (stapes). The eustachian tube, which reaches from the middle ear to the nasopharynx, allows for equalization of air pressure between this area and the outside, but unhappily, it may also serve as a source of infection to the middle ear. At the junction between the middle and inner ear, the vibrations are picked up by a membrane called the *oval window* and are

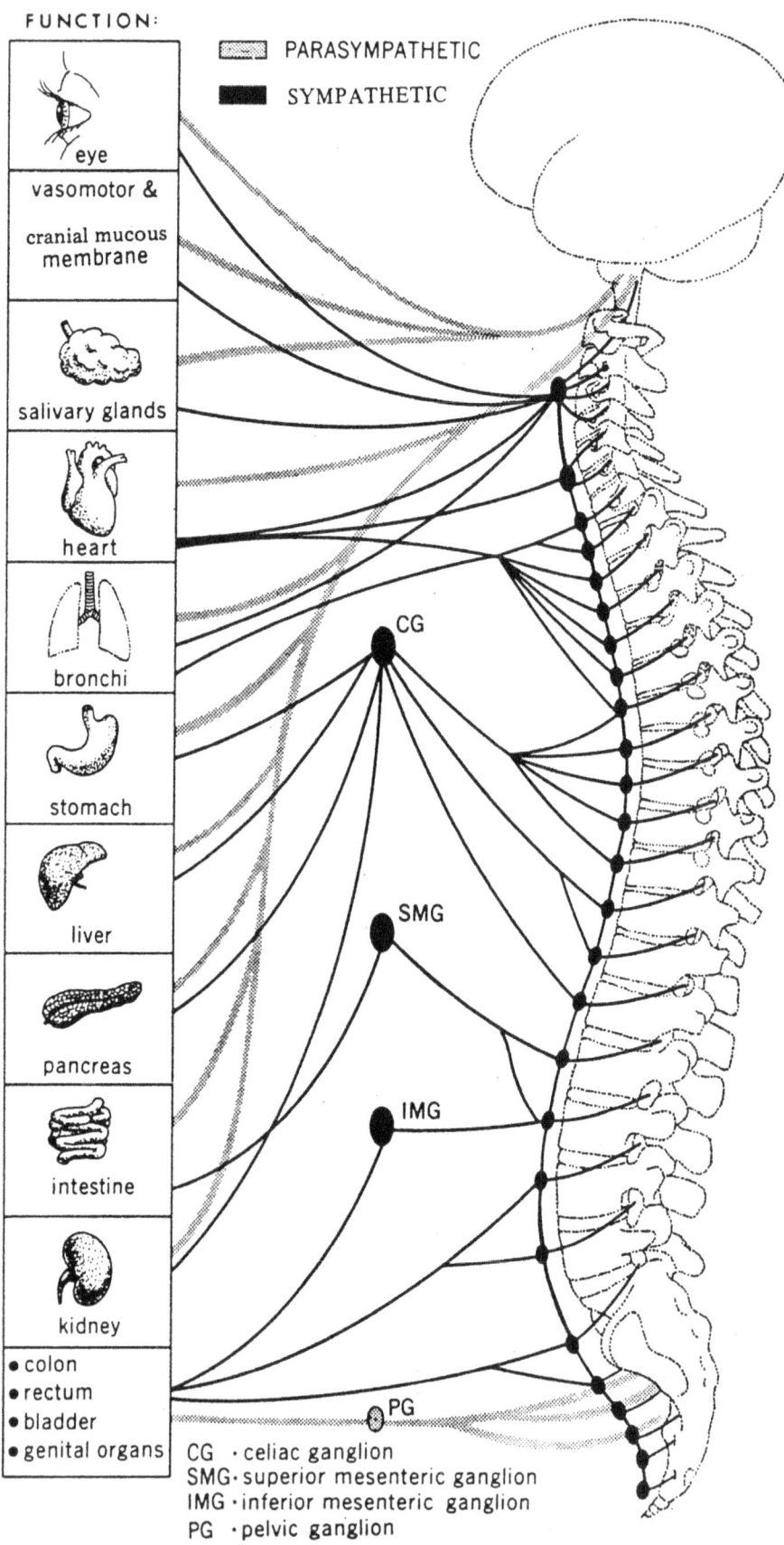

Figure 22. Diagram of the Autonomic Nervous System.

transferred through a fluid medium along the *cochlea*. The auditory (eighth cranial) nerve is stimulated by way of tiny hair cells (*organs of Corti*) which project into this fluid. The impulse is then carried to the auditory area of the brain, and hearing occurs. In addition to the cochlea, the inner ear also contains the semicircular canals. The fibers of the eighth cranial nerve, which controls equilibrium, reach into this organ and pick up messages which inform us of the position of our head. (In other words, this is where dizziness originates.)

d. The last two sensory organs, those of *smell* and *taste*, are closely allied. The nasal cavity contains the receptors of the *olfactory* (first cranial) nerve, and drawing air into the nose stimulates these nerve fibers. There are many kinds of smell receptors, and they fatigue easily as evidenced by how rapidly we become accustomed to any specific type of odor. *There are only four types of taste buds*, capable of stimulation by sweet, sour, bitter, or salty substances. The other flavors which we experience result from a combination of taste and smell.

SECTION E—THE CIRCULATORY SYSTEM

32. Functions of the Circulatory System. The circulatory system includes all structures concerned with the transportation and distribution of body fluids. It includes a *cardiovascular system* and a *lymphatic system*. These systems are vital to all other body systems and functions. The cardiovascular system consists of the heart, arteries, arterioles, veins, venules, and capillaries. The lymphatic system is made up of lymph capillaries, lymph vessels, and lymph ducts.

33. The Heart. Figure 26 illustrates the layers of the heart muscle, the four chambers, the valves dividing these chambers, and the manner in which major blood vessels lead into and out of the chambers. Coronary vessels nourish the heart muscle, and branches of the autonomic nervous system supply the impulses that cause the chambers to contract. One of the most common phenomenon associated with heart contractions is the *pulse*. The speed with which the heart contracts produces the *pulse rate*, and the force that blood exerts against the vessel walls with each contraction is *blood pressure*.

34. Circulation. The heart forces blood that has been freshly oxygenated by the lungs through *arterial* vessels, as illustrated in figure 27, to the *capillaries* that feed the cells of the body. *Veins*, shown in figure 28, then return the waste materials from the body cells to the heart, and the process is repeated.

35. Subdivisions of Blood. The two main subdivisions of blood are its *plasma* (liquid portion) and *formed elements*. Facts concerning this group of elements are contained in table 5, and the constituents of plasma are outlined in table 6. There are also certain elements which, by their presence or absence, determine *blood group* and *Rh factor*. The four blood groups are O, A, B, and AB. The Rh factor is indicated as negative (−) or positive (+). Both the blood group and Rh factor are important when a blood transfusion is to be given to a patient. If the blood of the donor and recipient are not compatible, severe reactions may occur which could endanger the life of the recipient.

36. The Lymphatic System. The lymphatic system, illustrated in figure 29, is discussed along with the circulatory system because the two systems

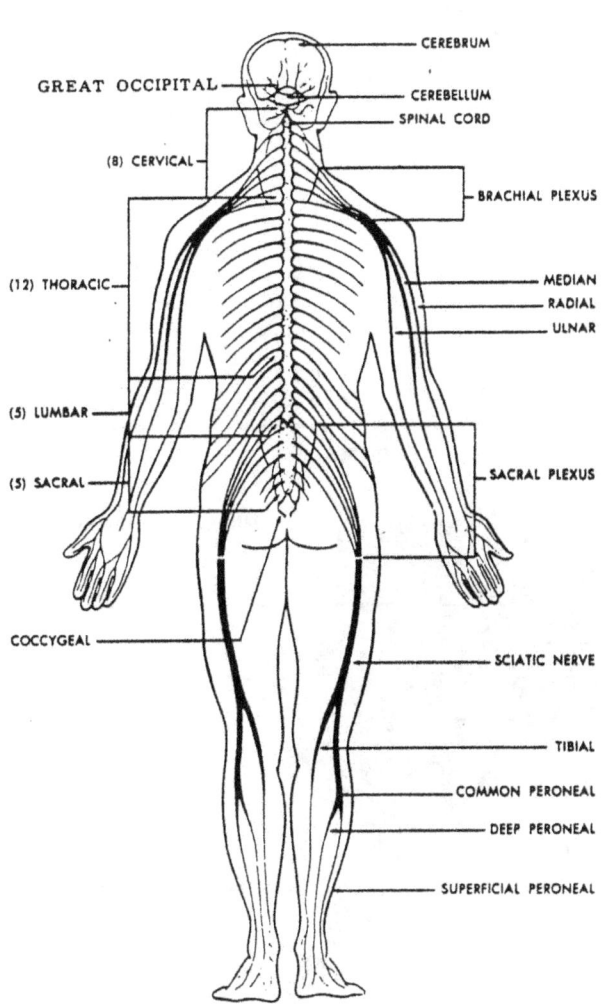

Figure 23. Major Nerve Branches of the Body.

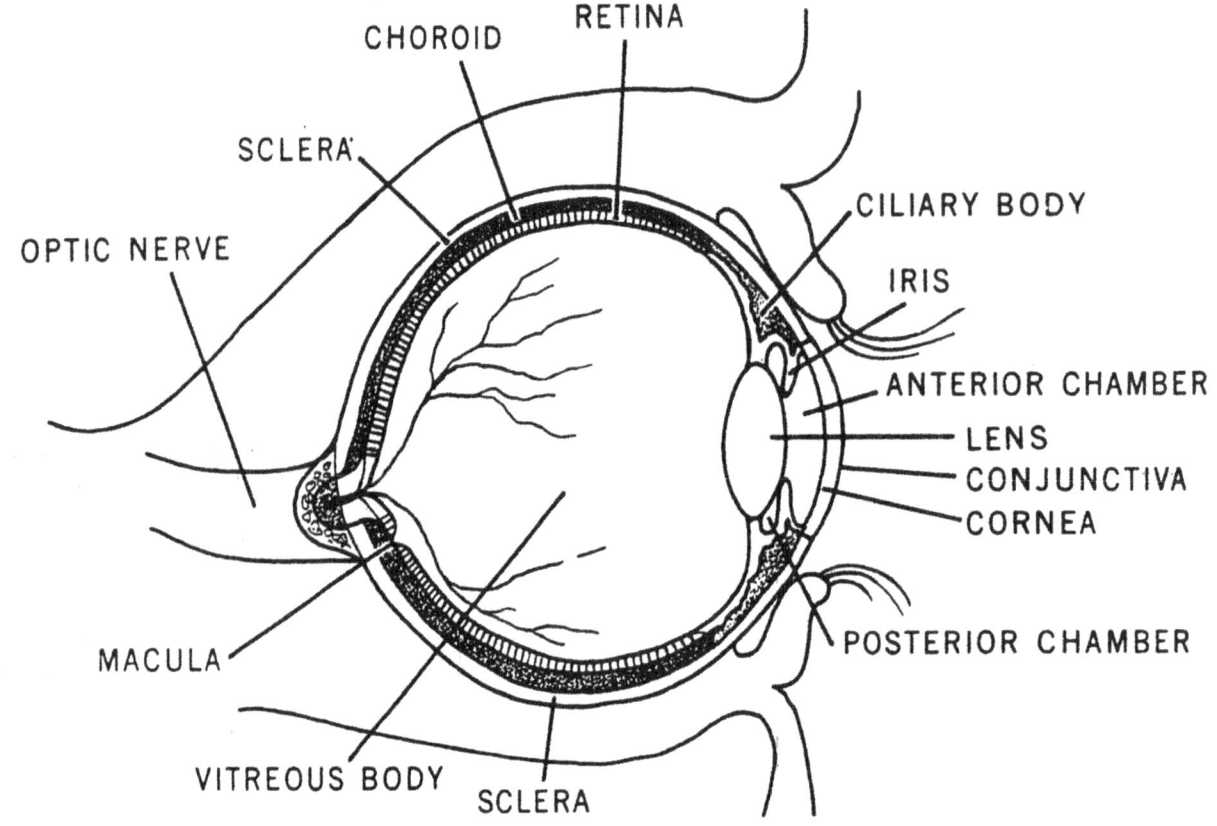

Figure 24. The Eye.

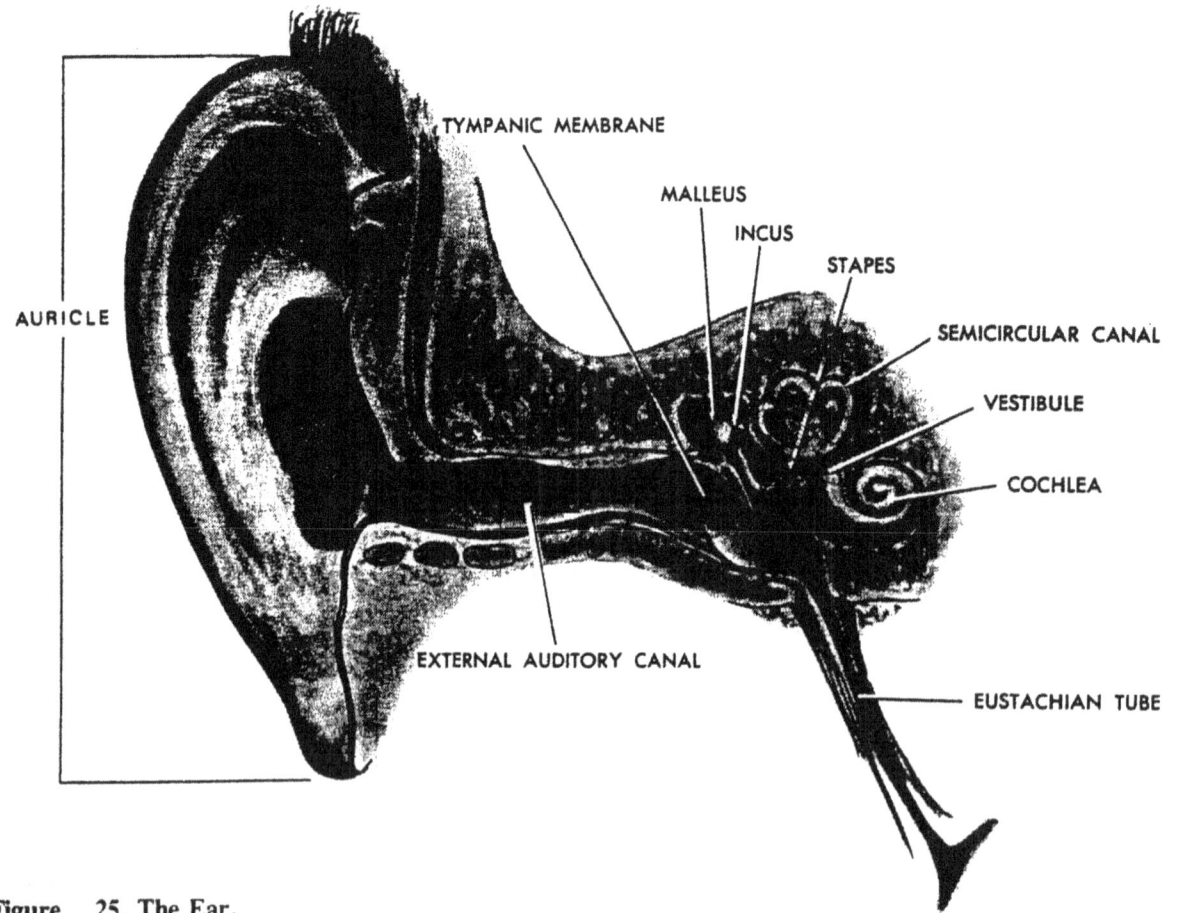

Figure 25. The Ear.

are closely associated. Lymphatic capillaries lie beneath the blood capillaries and collect fluid from the spaces between the cells. When lymph (tissue fluid) enters the lymphatic vessels it carries with it any bacteria that may have invaded these cells. Then, as this lymph proceeds through the lymphatic vessels, these bacteria are filtered out by *lymph nodes* and are destroyed by the action of lymphocytes. The lymph continues on into the main lymph ducts which empty into the neck veins.

SECTION F—THE RESPIRATORY SYSTEM

37. Function of the Respiratory System. The respiratory system includes the structures that are concerned with the exchange of gases (oxygen and carbon dioxide). The exchange of gases is known as respiration or breathing. It involves taking air into the lungs to obtain oxygen in exchange for carbon dioxide which is exhaled. It also involves the exchange of gases at the cellular level. The body requires a constant supply and exchange of these gases to carry on the chemical processes which are vital to life. Figure 30 illustrates the lungs and upper respiratory tract.

38. Anatomy of the Respiratory System. The respiratory system is composed of the nose, pharynx, larynx, trachea, lungs, bronchi, and pleurae. Accessory organs that make breathing possible are the thorax, ribs, diaphragm, and intercostal muscles.

a. *The Nose.* The *nose* is a framework of bone and cartilage with an external covering of skin. The

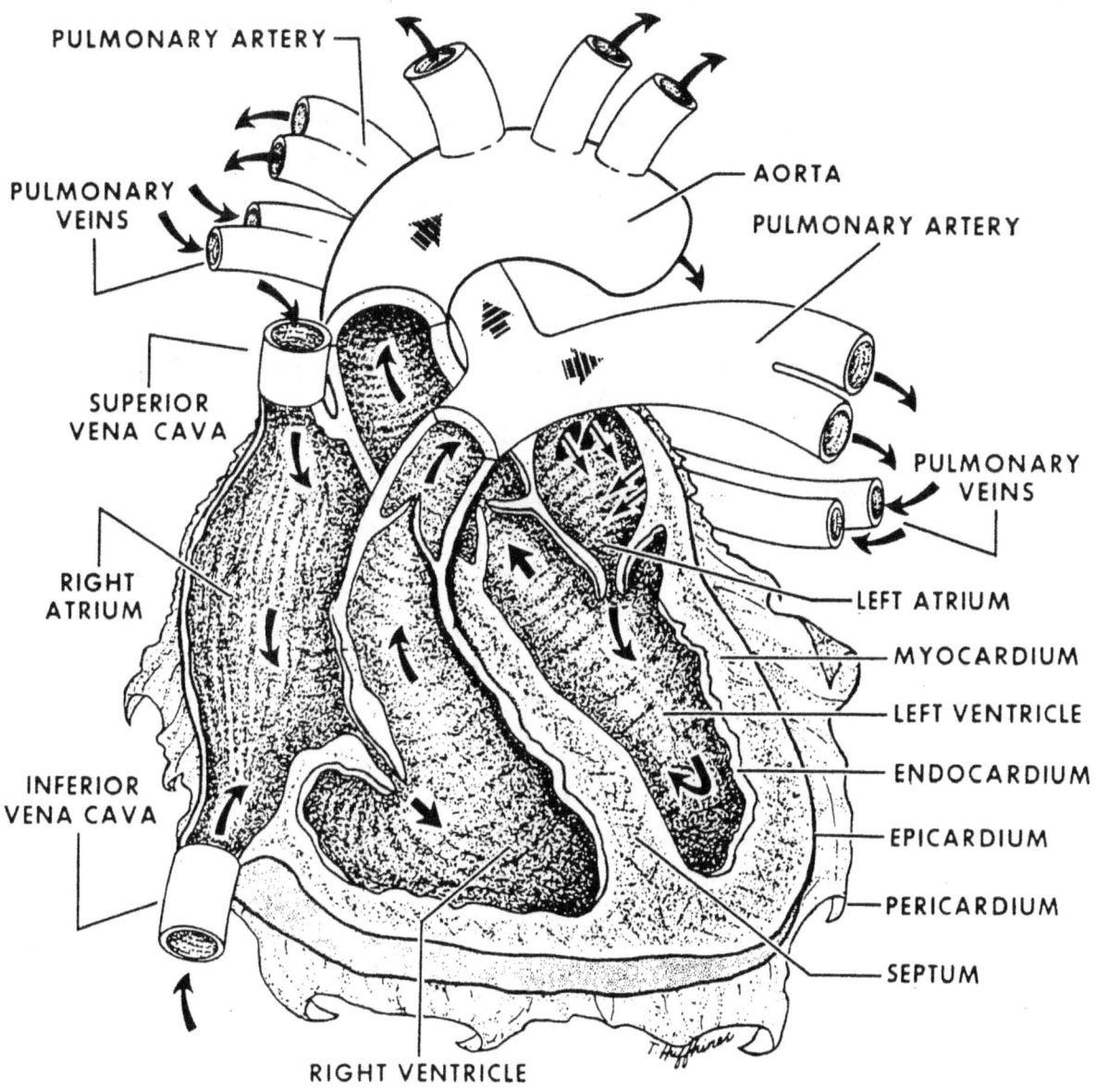

Figure 26. The Heart.

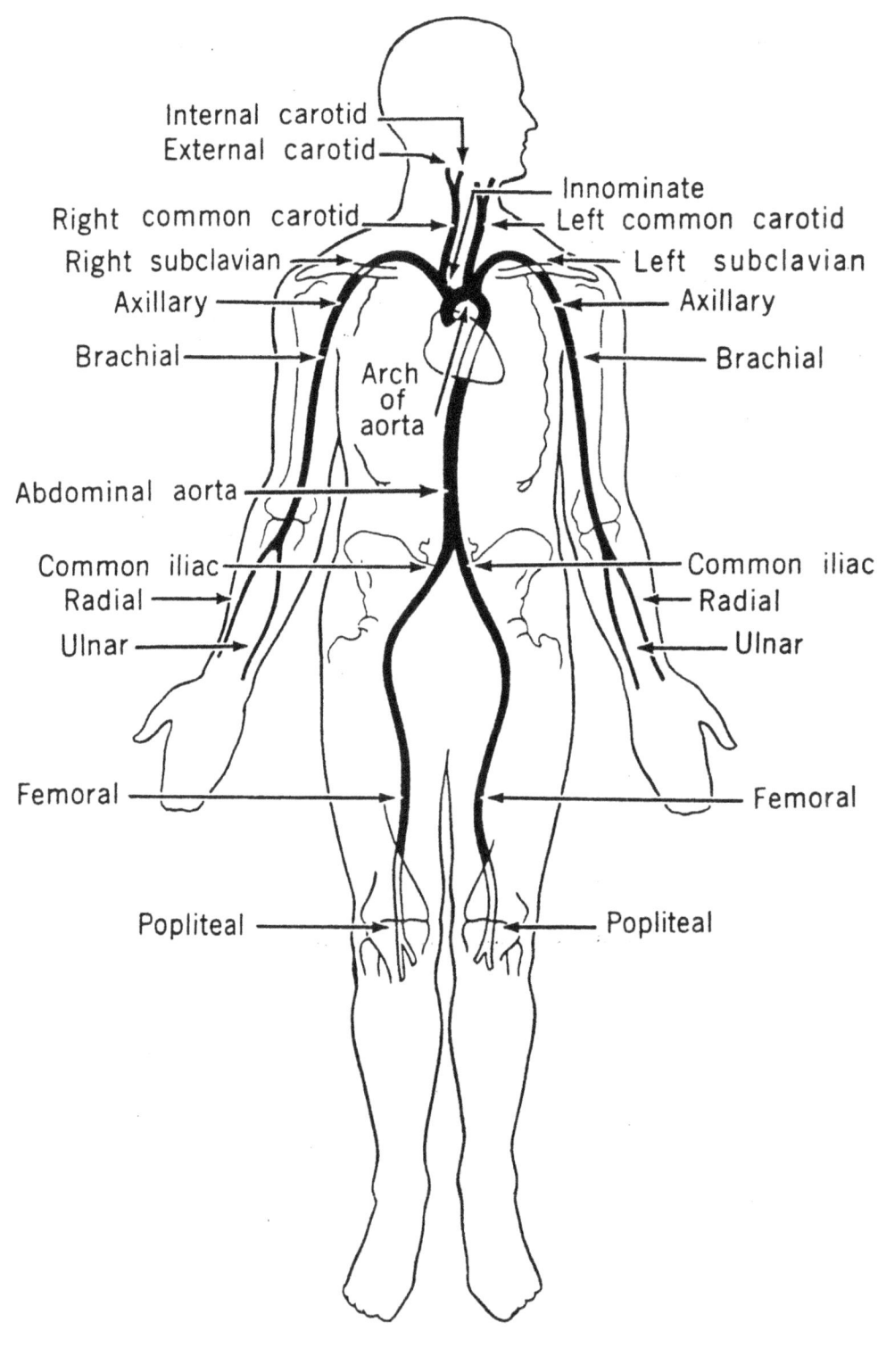

Figure 27. Major Arteries.

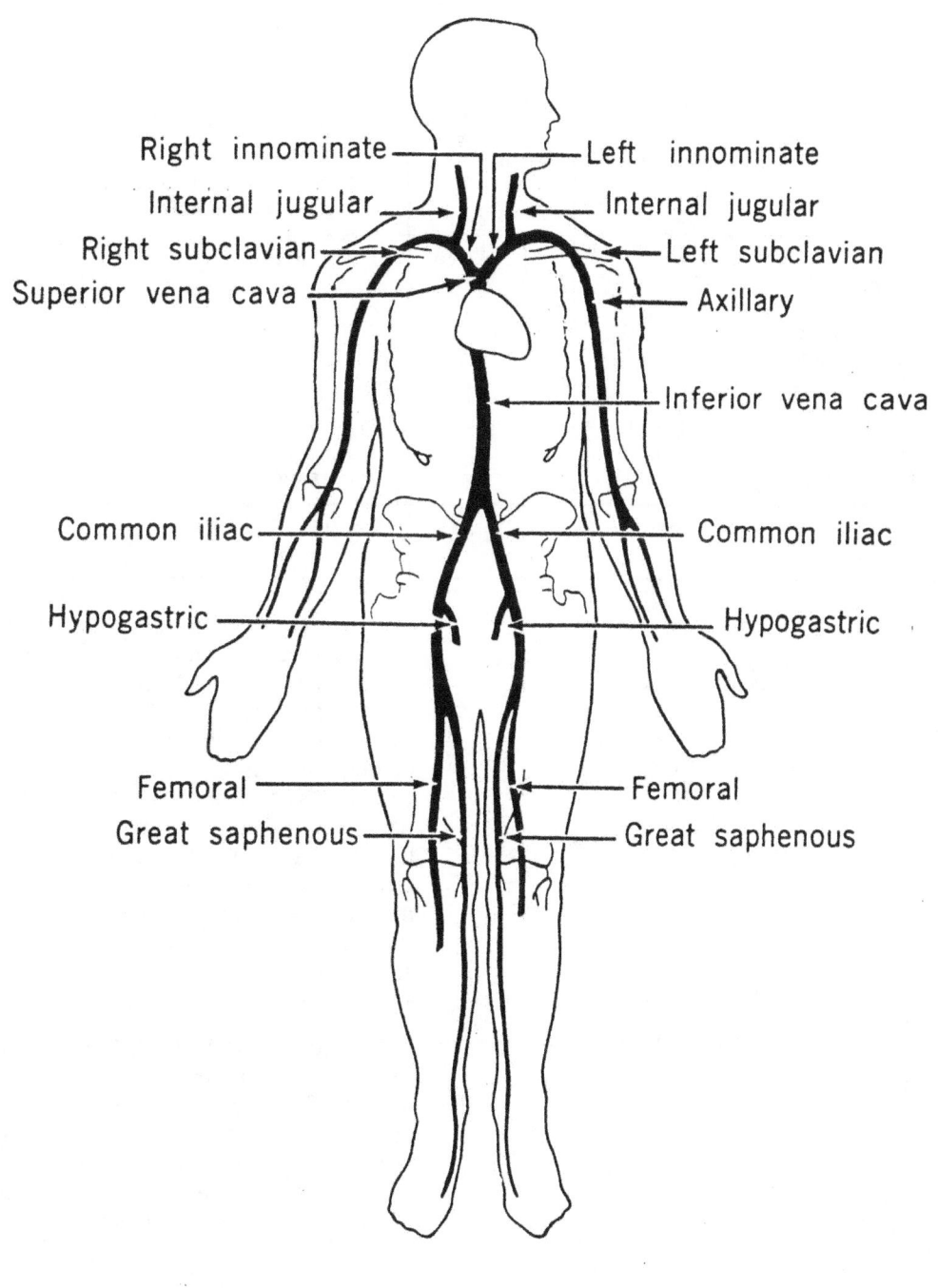

Figure 28. Major Veins.

Table 5. Formed Elements of Blood.

FORMED ELEMENTS OF BLOOD

Element	Source	Area of Destruction	Function
1. Erythrocytes (red cells)	Bone Marrow	Spleen, Liver	Respiration: Hemoglobin portion carries oxygen to cells and carbon dioxide away.
2. Leucocytes (white cells) Granulocytes: Neutrophils Eosinophils Basophils Agranulocytes: Lymphocytes Monocytes	Bone Marrow Lymph Nodes Unknown	Spleen, Liver	Fight infection Fight infection Form scar tissue, Some antibody formation
3. Thrombocytes (platelets)	Bone Marrow	Blood Clots	Coagulation of blood

Table 6. Constituents of Plasma.

CONSTITUENTS OF PLASMA

Substance	Purpose
Water (90% of blood volume)	Regulation of body temperature. Acts as solvent carrying substances to and from cells.
Proteins: Albumin	Buffer; regulates osmotic pressure
Globulin	Immunity
Fibrinogen	Blood clotting
Food: Glucose Amino acids Fat	Nourishment of the body
Vitamins Inorganic Salts: $+$ions $\quad$ $-$ions sodium $\quad$ chlorides potassium $\quad$ carbonates calcium $\quad$ bicarbonates magnesium $\quad$ sulfates iron $\quad$ phosphates $\quad$ iodides	Metabolism: Acid-base balance Osmosis Water distribution throughout body Irritability in muscles and nerves
Gases: Oxygen Carbon dioxide Nitrogen	Respiration
Hormones	Regulation of body functions
Enzymes	Digestion
Antibodies	Immunity to diseases
Waste products	To rid the body of unnecessary products of cell metabolism.

two external openings are called nostrils. They form the nasal cavity, which is divided into two parts by the nasal septum and separated from the mouth by the palate. The roof of the nasal cavity is formed from bones of the skull and face and is lined with mucous membrane. As air passes through the nasal cavity, it is warmed and moistened through contact with the mucous membrane. The air is also filtered; large foreign particles are caught by minute hairlike structures called cilia. The cilia cause wavelike movements of the particles from the anterior part of the nose to the pharynx. From here, these foreign particles are either expelled from the mouth or swallowed.

b. *The Pharynx.* The *pharynx* is the passageway between the nasal chambers, the nose, and the larynx. The *nasopharynx* is the superior portion of the pharynx and contains the two eustachian tubes which communicate with the middle ear. This provides an easy access for throat and nose infections to spread to the middle ear.

c. *The Larynx.* The *larynx*, or "voice box," is a passageway from the pharynx to the trachea. It is a triangular, cartilaginous structure composed of nine cartilages, joined together by ligaments. It lies in the middle of the neck, between the base of the tongue and the trachea. To prevent food from entering the trachea during the act of swallowing, the larynx moves upward and forward, placing it under the base of the tongue. This causes the epiglottis, a cartilaginous flap lying above the larynx, to move back and downward, directing the food into the esophagus. Knowing how this structure works becomes very important when caring for an unconscious or very ill patient. There is a danger that the

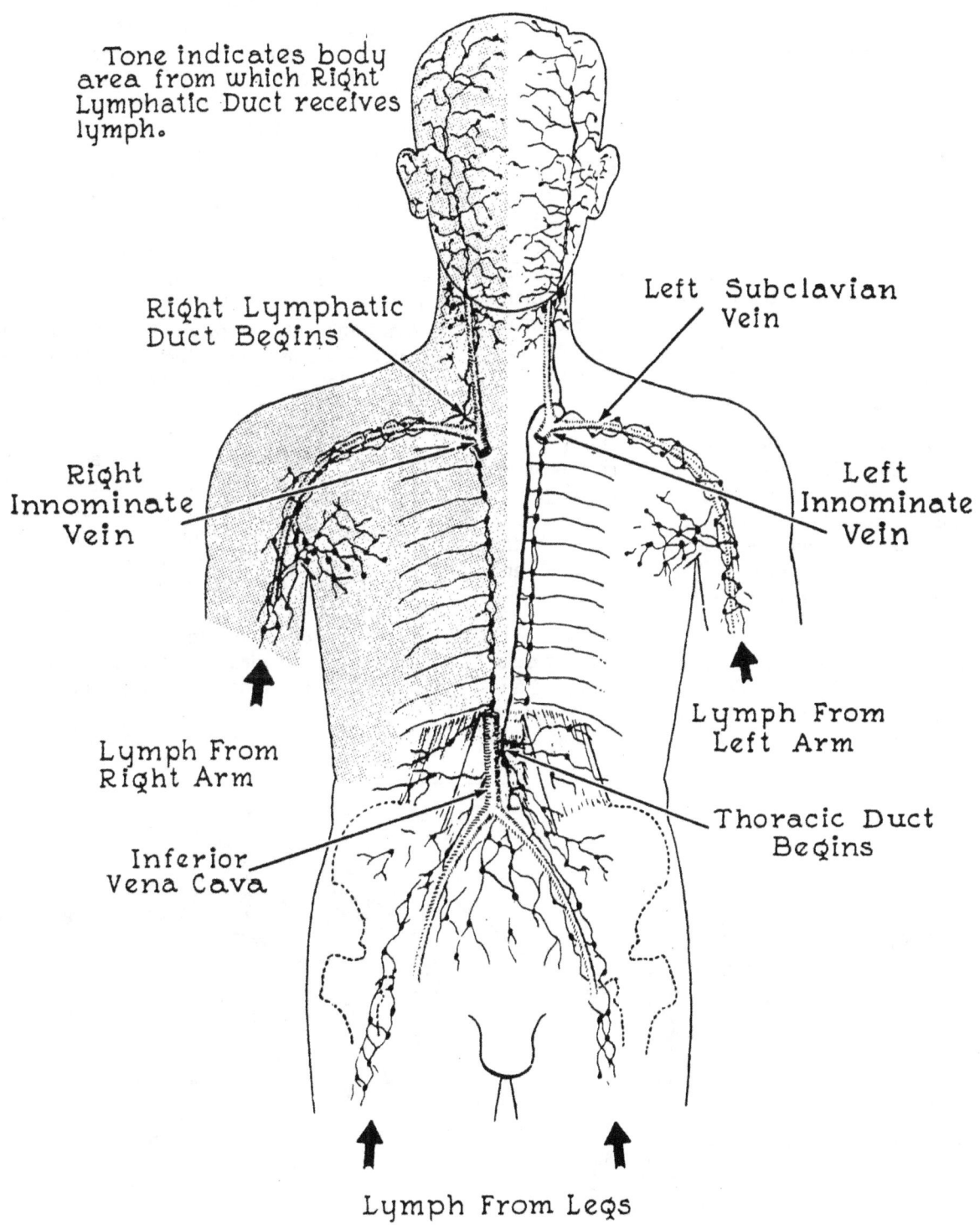

Figure 29. Lymphatic Vessels and Nodes.

tongue and pharyngeal tissues will relax and fall back into the oral pharynx, forcing the epiglottis down over the larynx. This causes obstruction of the airway. It can be relieved by pressing on the lower jaw and pushing it forward, keeping the teeth separated. On some occasions, it may be necessary to grasp the tongue and pull it forward. An artificial airway may be needed as an added precaution.

d. *The Trachea.* The *trachea* extends from the

larynx and terminates when it divides into the right and left bronchi. The trachea is lined with cilia and mucous glands which help entrap dust and foreign matter. The cilia beat upward, moving the particles to the larynx or pharynx, where they can be moved by coughing and expelled from the body.

e. *The Bronchi.* The trachea divides into *two primary bronchi* which convey air from the trachea to the lungs. After entering the lungs, each bronchus divides and sends branches to each lobe of the lungs: three to the right lung and two to the left lung. From here, they further divide into many small branches called bronchioles. These bronchioles go to the alveoli, or air sacs, of the lungs. The alveoli are adapted for easy passage of gases to and from the lung capillaries.

f. *The Lungs.* The *lungs* are the primary organs of respiration. They permit the interchange of gases between the blood and the air. The lungs are contained inside the thoracic cavity and enclosed in the pleurae. The *right lung contains three lobes;* the *left lung contains two lobes.* The lungs are soft and spongy and are constantly changing their form with each respiratory movement.

g. *Diffusion.* *Diffusion* is the equalization of gases (oxygen and carbon dioxide) between the blood and air. This process takes place in the lungs. Each lung contains thousands of tiny alveoli with blood capillaries in their membrane lining. Here oxygen is theoretically exchanged for carbon dioxide. This exchange also takes place between the capillaries and the tissues of the body. Oxygen cannot be stored by the lung or body tissue, so there is a continuous equalization or exchange of gases. Inhaled air contains about 20 percent oxygen and 0.03 percent carbon dioxide. Exhaled air contains about 16 percent oxygen and 4 percent carbon dioxide.

h. *Pleurae.* The lungs are enclosed in double-walled, serous membranes called the pleurae. Each lung has a separate pleura. The membrane or sac covering the outer surface of the lung is called the visceral layer, and the other layer lining the chest wall is called the parietal layer. The area between these two membranes is called the intrathoracic or pleural space. However, this is only a potential space since the pleural membranes are in very close contact with one another. The only substance separating them is a small amount of pleural fluid, secreted by the membrane. This pleural fluid reduces friction between the two pleural layers during the movements of respiration. Without this fluid a condition known as "dry pleurisy" results, occurring most often in pneumonia. It results in pain because the two pleural membranes rub together (friction fremitus) during each respiration.

i. *The Diaphragm and Intercostal Muscles.* The

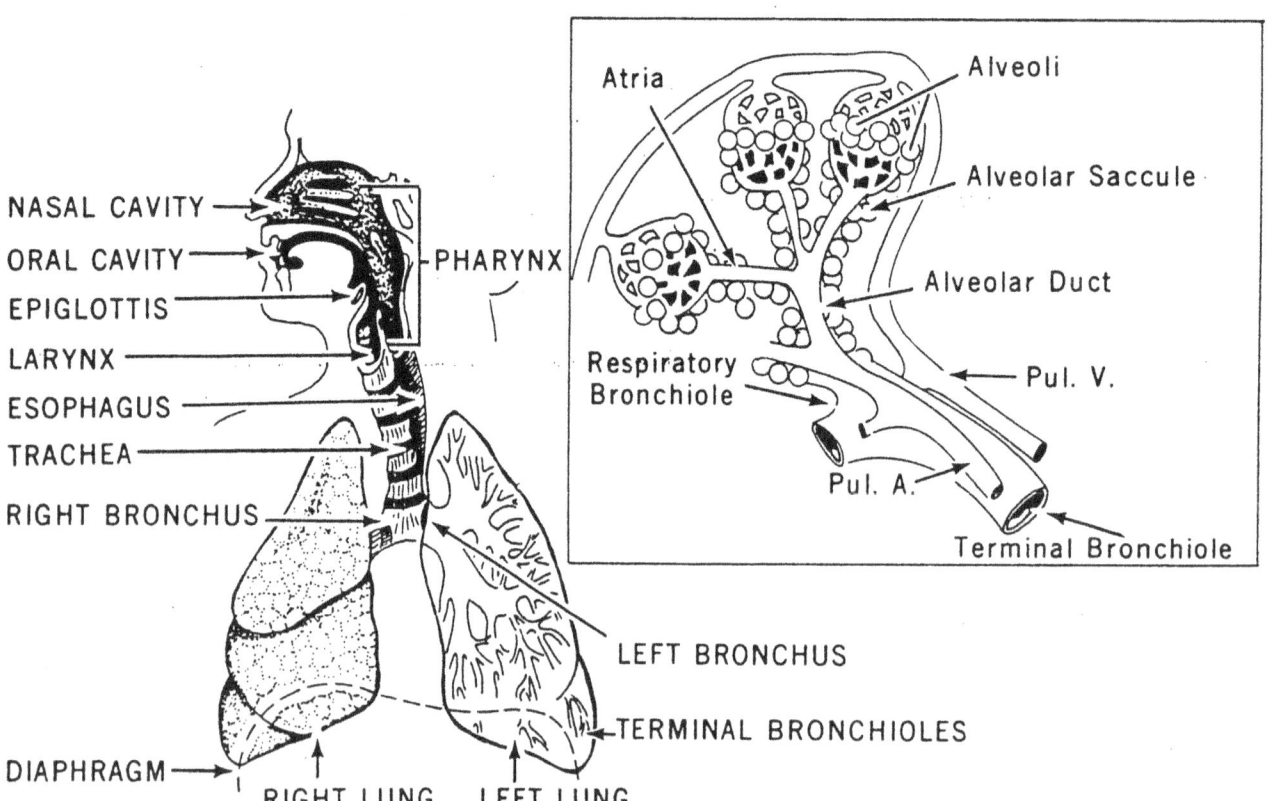

Figure 30. Schematic Drawing of the Lungs and Upper Respiratory Tract.

simple *process of breathing* (inspiration and expiration) is far more complex than it first appears. It is a harmonious interplay of nerve impulses, muscular activity, and mechanical pressure changes, which are all influenced by chemical changes in the blood. The inflation of the lungs occurs because the muscles of respiration contract. These muscles are the *diaphragm* and the *intercostal muscles*.

j. Inspiration and Expiration. In the act of *inspiration*, the intercostal muscles contract and help to enlarge the size of the thorax; the ribs move forward and slightly upward, increasing the front-to-back dimensions of the thorax. There is a slight increase in the side-to-side dimensions at the same time. This mechanical change, combined with the downward movement of the diaphragm, enlarges the thorax and produces a pressure decrease in the intrathoracic space—the potential space between the surface of the lungs and the internal lining of the thorax. Since the lungs are inside the thorax, and the interior of the lungs is exposed to the atmospheric pressure outside the body, atmospheric pressure forces air through the conducting passages and into the alveoli. When inspiration is complete, the muscles of inspiration relax, and because of the elasticity of the chest wall and the lungs, expiration occurs.

39. Breathing. Breathing is normally an *involuntary* act controlled by the nervous system. A diffuse group of nerve cells known collectively as the respiratory center is located in the medulla oblongata (brain). The nerve impulses, which cause the muscles of respiration to contract, originate in the cells of the respiratory center. These impulses reach the respiratory muscles by two sets of nerves—the *phrenic nerves* and the *intercostal nerves*. The phrenic nerves pass down into the thorax to the diaphragm. The intercostal nerves leave the spinal cord in the upper region of the back and pass to the intercostal muscles. Nerve impulses from the walls of the alveoli return to the respiratory center through two *vagus nerves* which pass upward through the thorax and neck to the medulla. When the lungs inflate and the walls of the alveoli are stretched to the maximum for the needs of the body at that particular time, nerve impulses return to the respiratory center and stop the impulses to the muscles of inspiration. Passive expiration then follows. This continuing process of inspiration and expiration is primarily involuntary and continues even though a person is asleep or unconscious. There is a degree of *conscious control over breathing*, however. For example, it is possible for a person to hold his or her breath, and it is also possible for the conscious will to control the rate and depth of breathing. This control is from a high voluntary center of the brain in the cerebral cortex.

Impulses from these higher centers reach the involuntary respiratory center over specific nerve pathways and temporarily override its automatic function. Nerve impulses from it, then, are in accordance with the desires of the higher center. This control by the higher center is limited by chemical changes in the blood which will occur in time, and the control then reverts back to the involuntary center.

SECTION G—THE DIGESTIVE SYSTEM

40. The Alimentary Canal. The digestive system is divided into two separate divisions—the *alimentary canal* and the *accessory organs of digestion*. The entire system includes all of the organs concerned with the ingestion of food, its absorption, and the nutrition of body cells.

a. The Mouth. The mouth contains the *salivary glands*, the *teeth*, and the *tongue*, as illustrated in figure 31. The salivary glands are accessory digestive glands. The teeth aid in the digestive process by masticating food. The tongue is a muscular organ closely associated with the function of taste, mastication, salivation, and swallowing.

b. The Stomach. The stomach, shown in figure 32, is a saccular enlargement of the gastrointestinal tract which stores and digests food. It is located in the upper left quadrant of the abdomen just below the diaphragm. Two muscular rings or sphincters guard the entrance to, and the exit from, the stomach. The *cardiac sphincter* at the upper end of the stomach opens and allows food to enter from the esophagus, and the *pyloric sphincter* at the lower end controls the entry of food into the duodenum (the beginning of the small intestine).

(1) Numerous tiny glands in the stomach secrete gastric juice containing enzymes and hydrochloric acid. This gastric juice starts protein digestion. The hydrochloric acid also acts as a disinfectant to destroy any bacteria which may have been taken in with the food. Food remains in the stomach for 3 to 4 hours while peristalsis churns and thoroughly mixes the food with the gastric juices. The result is a semiliquid substance called chyme.

(2) Chyme is released through the pyloric sphincter into the duodenum, where further digestion takes place. Some drugs, a small amount of water, concentrated sugar, and alcohol are absorbed by the stomach, all in small amounts.

c. The Small Intestine. The small intestine is a much-coiled muscular tube about 20 feet long. It consists of three parts: the *duodenum*, the *jejunum*, and the *ileum*.

(1) The duodenum is lined with glands which secrete intestinal juices. The bile and pancreatic ducts open into the duodenum, as noted in figure 33.

(2) The jejunum, extending from the duodenum to the ileum, is the middle segment of the small intestine. Minor food absorption takes place here.

(3) The majority of food absorption takes place in the ileum. It is lined with fingerlike processes called villi, which provide a larger absorption area. The villi also contain lymph channels and a network of blood capillaries. After food has been digested, it is absorbed into the capillaries and lymph channels and carried to all parts of the body. Material that cannot be digested and absorbed passes through the ileocecal valve into the large intestine.

d. *The Large Intestine.* The large intestine, often called the colon, consists of the cecum, ascending colon, transverse colon, descending colon, sigmoid colon, and the rectum. The large intestine is about 5 feet in length and about 2 inches in diameter. It absorbs water from the liquid contents it receives.

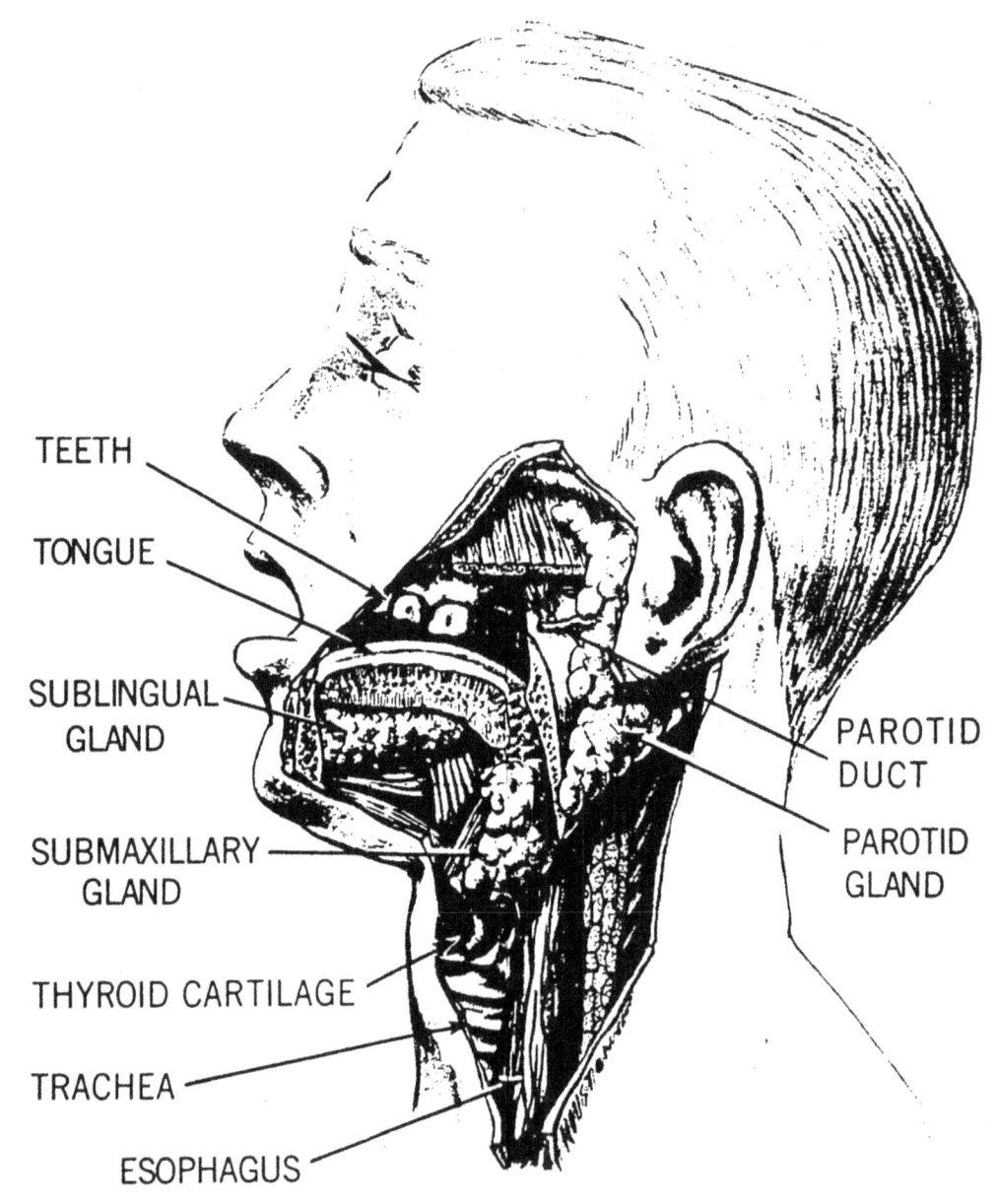

Figure 31. Upper Alimentary Tract.

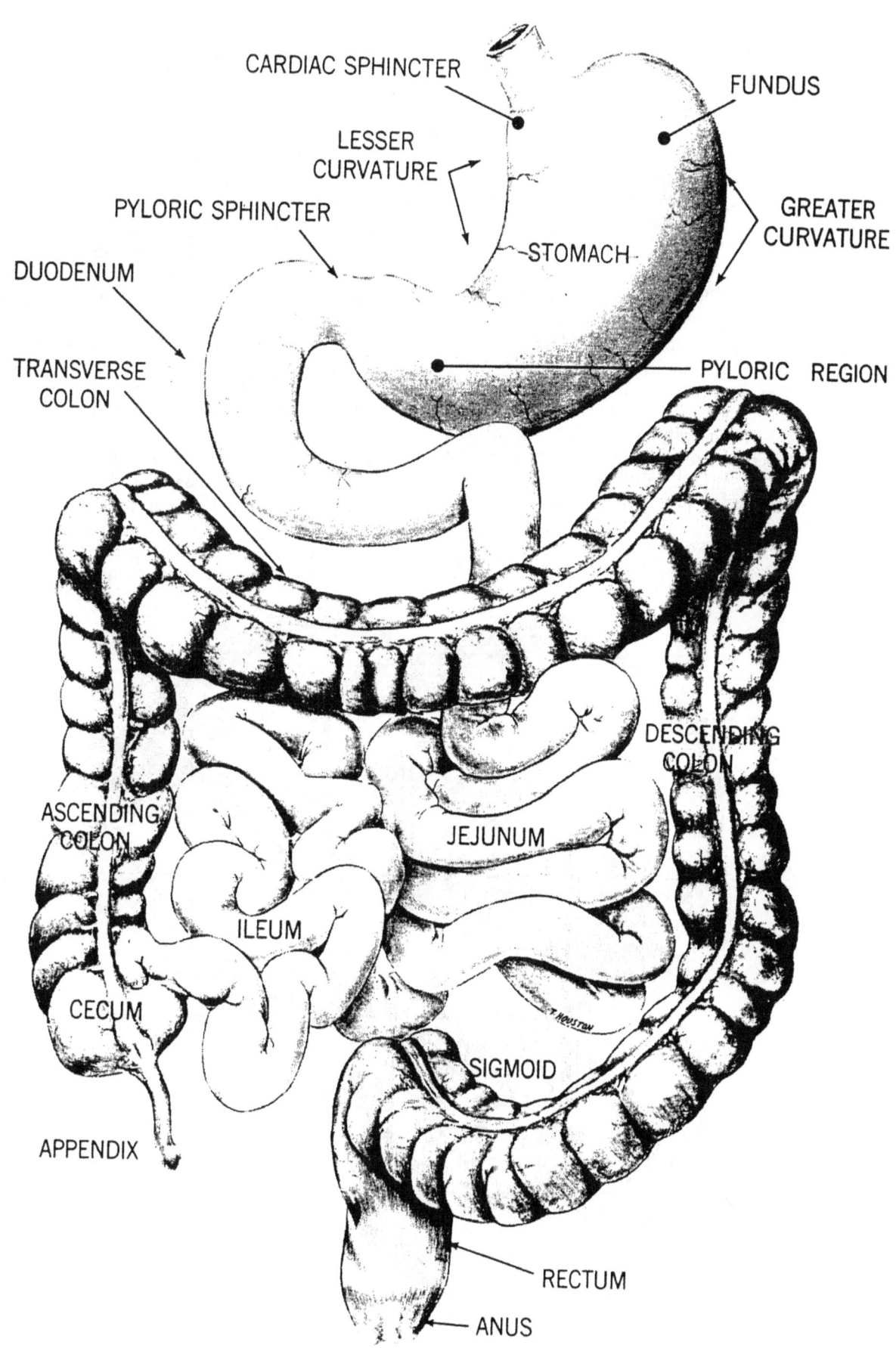

Figure 32. Stomach and Intestines.

Glands in its walls secrete mucus, which mixes with the remaining material and helps form the stool or feces.

41. The Accessory Organs of Digestion. The accessory organs of digestion, illustrated in figure 33, include the liver, gallbladder, pancreas, and the salivary glands.

  a. *The Liver.* The liver is one of the largest glands in the body; it is located in the right upper quadrant of the abdomen just below the diaphragm. It is a very vascular gland and is divided into lobes. Each lobe has a duct for collecting bile. The ducts join together in each lobe and leave the liver as the hepatic duct. The hepatic artery and vein furnish a rich supply of blood to the liver. All blood from the stomach and small intestines passes through the liver by means of the portal vein. The liver not only *aids in digestion,* it also *aids in the metabolism of carbohydrates, proteins, and fats; helps maintain the proper level of sugar in the blood; produces heparin and fibrinogen which influence the clotting of blood; and detoxifies substances which might be harmful to the human body.*

  b. *The Gallbladder.* The duct system of the liver transports bile from the liver cells to the duodenum or to the gallbladder for storage. The gallbladder is a reservoir for concentrating and storing bile. It is about 3 to 4 inches long and has a capacity of about 50 cm^3. It is shaped somewhat like a blackjack and is located in a hollow on the underside of the liver. Its duct, the cystic duct, joins the hepatic duct from the liver to form the common bile duct, which enters the duodenum at the ampulla of Vater. When food arrives in the duodenum, the gallbladder contracts and bile is sent through the cystic duct into the common bile duct and into the duodenum.

  c. *The Pancreas.* The pancreas is a long gland with its body or main part lying below the liver and the stomach, and adjacent to the duodenum. Its "tail" extends transversely to the left and terminates near the spleen. The pancreas provides pancreatic juice and the hormone, insulin.

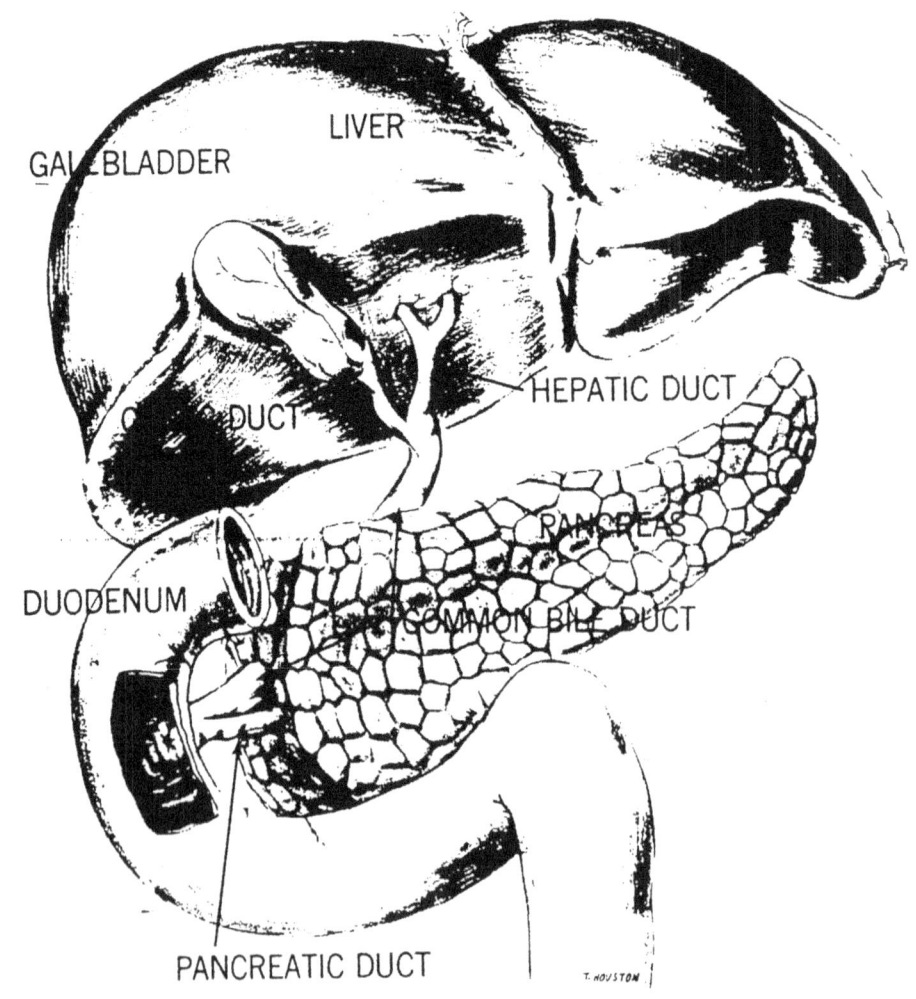

Figure 33. Accessory Organs of Digestion.

d. *The Salivary Glands.* The salivary glands are located in the mouth and are named according to their location.

42. Effect of the Nervous System. The digestive process is also affected by the nervous system. For example, sympathetic impulses that speed up the heart rate and respiratory rate will slow the digestive process. This phenomenon is often evident when a patient has sustained injuries in an accident. Because of the excitement, the digestive processes are delayed, and the stomach may remain filled with undigested food for a long period of time. If the patient is given general anesthetic, the anesthetist must be constantly alert for vomiting as *the anesthetized patient is unable to swallow.* Therefore, any vomitus might be drawn into the trachea and result in suffocation.

SECTION H—THE ENDOCRINE SYSTEM

43. The Glands of Internal Secretion. The endocrine system is composed of the *glands of internal secretion.* They are called ductless and internal glands because they have no ducts to carry away their secretions. Their secretions enter directly into the blood or lymph circulation and eventually reach the organ or organs which they influence or control. Very small quantities of hormones are produced with only a small amount necessary to produce an effect. Some hormones may influence only one part of the body, while others influence the body as a whole. The hormone-producing glands are the pituitary, thyroid, parathyroid, adrenals, pancreas, gonads, intestinal, the pineal body, and the thymus gland. These glands are shown in figure - 34.

a. The pituitary gland is a small gland that has a tremendous influence on the body. It is often referred to as the "master gland," since it has regulatory control over the functions of other glands. It has an *anterior* and a *posterior* lobe and secretes at least nine hormones. Hormones produced by the anterior lobe of the pituitary are growth, thyrotropic, gonadotropic, adrenocorticotropic, and lactogenic. Antidiuretic hormones, vasopressin, and oxytoxin are produced by the posterior lobe of the pituitary gland.

b. The thyroid gland (largest of the endocrine glands) is a butterfly-shaped gland lying in the anterior middle portion of the neck, just below the larynx. It consists of two lateral lobes united by a strip called the isthmus. It has an abundant blood supply furnished by branches of the external carotid and the subclavian arteries. It produces a hormone called thyroxin, which is about 65 percent iodine. Thyroxin performs many functions. It regulates the rate of oxidation and the heat production of the body; it is concerned with growth and differentiation of body organs; it plays a part in mental development; and indirectly affects sexual maturity. It also plays a part in the distribution and the exchange of water, salts, and proteins and has some influence in the production of glucose from amino acids.

c. The adrenal glands are sometimes called the suprarenal glands, since they lie like small caps on the top of each kidney. Each gland has two parts, the medulla and the cortex, and each part produces a different hormone.

(1) The medulla secretes *epinephrine* and norephrine. Epinephrine is one of the most powerful vasopressors known; it increases blood pressure, accelerates the heart muscle, and increases cardiac output. Epinephrine (adrenalin) is used as a cardiac stimulant, a pressor (increases blood pressure) substance, and to relax bronchial smooth muscles.

(2) The cortex secretes several hormones called *cortisones.* The cortex is stimulated by the pituitary hormone. *ACTH* (adrenocorticotropic hormone). Hormones secreted by the cortex help to regulate muscular activity, reproduction, salt metabolism, water electrolyte balance, and kidney function.

d. The pancreas is located behind the stomach and is a double-functioning gland; it produces secretions which are discharged into the duodenum (exocrine or duct gland) and insulin which is discharged into the blood stream (endocrine or ductless gland). *Insulin* is a hormone essential for the use and storage of carbohydrates by the body.

e. The gonads serve a double function in both sexes—the development of reproductive cells (ova and sperm) and the production of hormones.

(1) The principal hormone of the testes is *testosterone.* It regulates the development of secondary sex characteristics, such as hair on the chest and face, deeper voice, and general development of the male stature.

(2) The principal hormones of the female are *estrogen* and *progesterone.* Estrogen is responsible for the secondary sex characteristics, such as body form and development of the mammary glands. Progesterone is responsible for changes in the uterine lining during the second half of the menstrual cycle. It prepares the uterus for the implantation of the fertilized ovum, and for the development of the embryo in the early stages of its growth. It also supplements the action of estrogen on the mammary glands during pregnancy.

f. Other glands which must be considered are the intestinal, the pineal, and the thymus glands. The

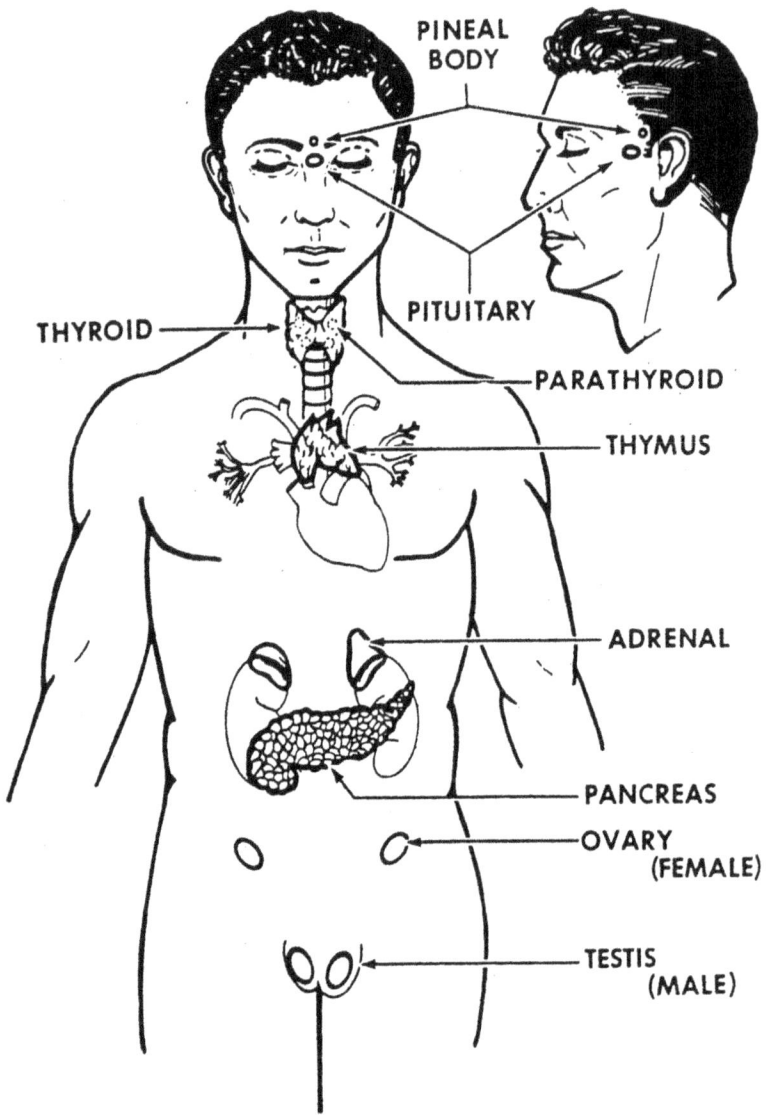

Figure 34. Locations and Approximate Locations of the Endocrine Glands.

intestinal glands secrete a hormone called secretin. Secretin stimulates the secretion of pancreatic juice and bile. The pineal gland is a small gland located within the midpoint of the brain. Its endocrine secretion and function are uncertain. The thymus gland lies within the midline of the chest cavity. Its function is also obscure.

44. The Effect of Endocrine Glands on Surgical Decisions. The functions of the endocrine glands have a decided effect on the decision of the surgeon to remove any one of these glands. If it is deemed necessary to remove the total gland, the doctor must consider the necessity of administering the hormone, originally produced by the gland, by artificial means. For this reason, the surgeon often removes only part of a gland and leaves intact any normal portion which he or she thinks will continue to secrete hormones.

45. Effect of the Endocrine Glands on General Health. Another problem which the surgeon must consider before undertaking procedures that don't actually involve the endocrine organs is that of malfunction of these organs to the extent that ordinary body processes cannot be properly maintained during or after an operative procedure. Treatment of an endocrine malfunction may be necessary before even routine surgery is undertaken.

SECTION I—THE URINARY SYSTEM

46. Anatomy of the Urinary System. The urinary system includes the organs that are concerned with the production and elimination of urine. This system consists of the kidneys, the ureters, the urinary bladder, and the urethra. These structures secrete and eliminate urine, a liquid waste product of cell metabolism. Figure 35 illustrates the structures of the urinary system.

a. *The Kidneys.* The kidneys are paired, bean-shaped organs, located on each side of the vertebral column, posterior to the abdominal cavity, at about the level of the 12th rib. Each is surrounded by fat and connective tissue, and enclosed in a fibrous-type capsule. Each kidney is about 1 inch thick, 2 inches wide, and 4 inches long. It weighs about 6 ounces. The right kidney is slightly lower than the left because of the position of the liver.

(1) The kidney is a highly complex organ with three important functions: to filter the blood, discarding materials no longer needed; to maintain water and electrolyte balance; and to maintain acid-base balance.

(2) Each kidney has two main layers. The outer layer, called the *cortex* and an inner layer called the *medulla*. The medulla contains a number of cone-shaped divisions called pyramids. These pyramids extend into the renal pelvis, which in turn, empties into the ureter.

(3) The artery and vein supplying each kidney are the *renal* artery and the renal vein. The renal artery comes directly from the abdominal aorta, and the renal vein enters the inferior vena cava.

(4) As blood flows through the kidneys, it is filtered and purified by nephron units. Each nephron unit consists of a series of tiny tubules. Each tubule extends from the capsule and joins with other tubules in the medulla region; it descends, loops, ascends, twists, and then terminates into a single collecting tube. The products of filtration pass through the collecting tubules into the funnel-shaped pyramids, to the calyces, and then to the renal pelvis, where they finally enter the ureters. These units are responsible for all the filtering, excreting, and reabsorbing that takes place within the kidneys. A cross section of a kidney is illustrated in figure 36.

b. *Urine.* The end product of kidney filtration is urine. Normally it is amber-colored, free of bacteria, and about 95 percent water. The other 5 percent is made-up of various organic and inorganic compounds. Under normal conditions, an adult excretes from 1500 to 2000 cm³ of urine in 24 hours. However, this amount can be influenced by such factors as body temperature, humidity, and fluid intake.

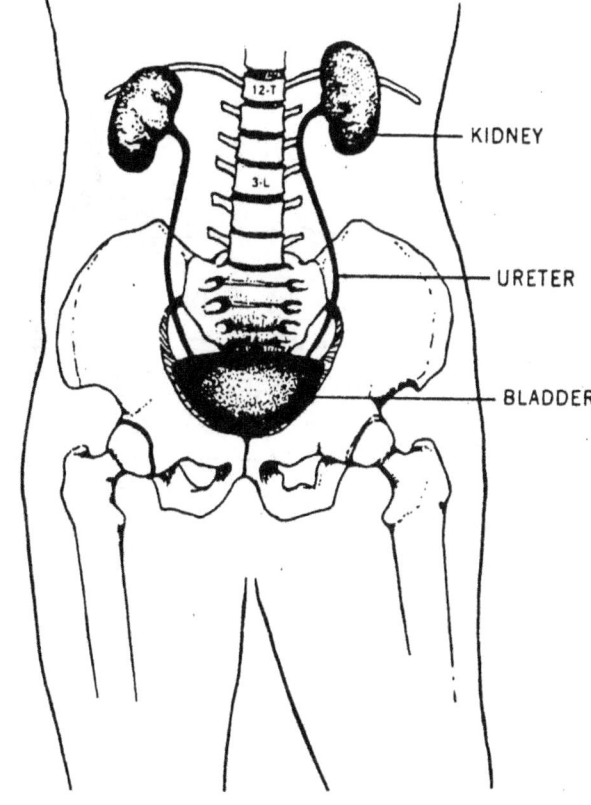

Figure 35. The Urinary System.

SECTION J—THE REPRODUCTIVE SYSTEM

47. Purpose of the Reproductive System. The primary purpose of the reproductive system is to allow for a union of male and female sex cells.

a. *Male Reproductive System.* The male organs of reproduction are the penis, testes, and the associated ducts and glands. The entire system is shown in figure 37.

(1) The *testes* are oval glands suspended by the spermatic cords in a cutaneous pouch, the scrotum. They perform two functions: production of spermatozoa and secretion of the male sex hormone, testosterone. Lying closely adjacent to the superior pole of each testis is the epididymis, a ductal system that collects and transmits sperm cells from the testis. The epididymis runs down the length of the testicle, then turns upward as a straight tube and becomes the vas deferens.

(2) The *scrotum* is part of the male external genitalia. It is a pouchlike sac containing the testes and a part of the spermatic cord. The scrotum, hanging between the legs, exposes the testes to a temperature lower than that of the body, which is

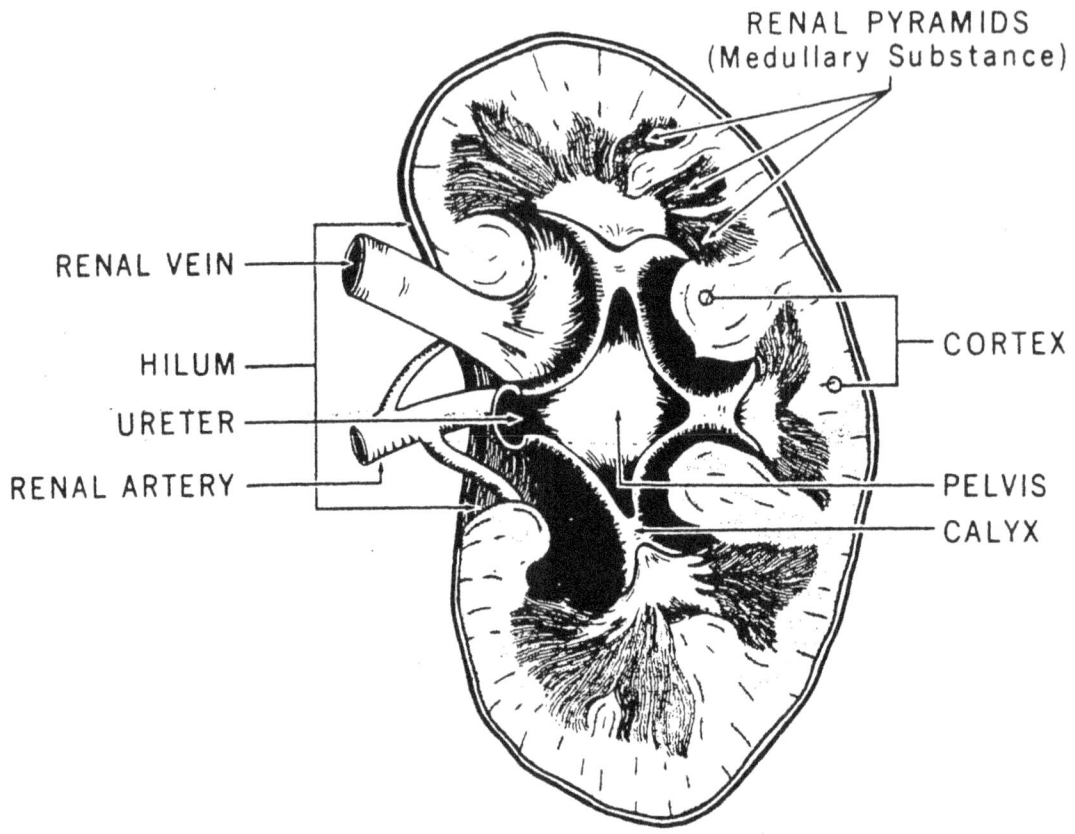

Figure 36. Cross Section of Kidney.

essential for proper development of sperm. Occasionally, a child is born with the testes undescended. This condition, called cryptorchidism, is corrected by surgery.

(3) Two *spermatic cords* each of which suspends and supplies a testis, are formed by the *vas deferens*, spermatic artery, vein, lymphatic vessels, and nerves, and are bound together by connective tissue.

(4) The *vas deferens* (ductus deferens) is a small convoluted tube about 2 feet long that carries sperm cells from the epididymis to the seminal vesicle. There they join and form the ejaculatory duct.

(5) The *seminal vesicles* are two pouches that lie just above the prostate, between the bladder and the rectum. They secrete seminal fluid and serve as a storage place for testicular secretion which is expelled at the time of ejaculation.

(6) The vas deferens and the duct from the seminal vesicles converge and form the ejaculatory duct which leads into the prostatic urethra. Testicular secretion is forced through the ejaculatory duct into the urethra by muscle contraction.

(7) The *prostate gland* is made-up of the smooth muscle and granular tissue that surrounds the proximal portion of the urethra. It resembles a chestnut in size and shape, and secretes an alkaline fluid into the urethra during ejaculation. This fluid keeps the sperm mobile and protects them from the acid secretions of the female vagina. The prostate gland can also be the source of considerable trouble in later life. It has a tendency to enlarge, which may interfere with urination by shutting off the urethra. It also has a tendency to develop cancer and may be surgically removed. Removal is called a prostatectomy. Surgical removal can be accomplished by several different surgical approaches. The physician's choice usually depends upon the age of the patient, the reason for the removal, and the size of the prostate gland.

b. *Female Reproductive System.* The female reproductive system, shown in figure 38, includes the ovaries, fallopian tubes, uterus, vagina, and external genitalia. Although the perineum and the mammary glands are not part of the system, they are clearly associated with its function.

(1) The *ovaries* are two almond-shaped glands that lie on each side of the uterus near the ends of the fallopian tubes. Connecting the ovaries to the uterus are the ovarian ligaments. The ovaries pro-

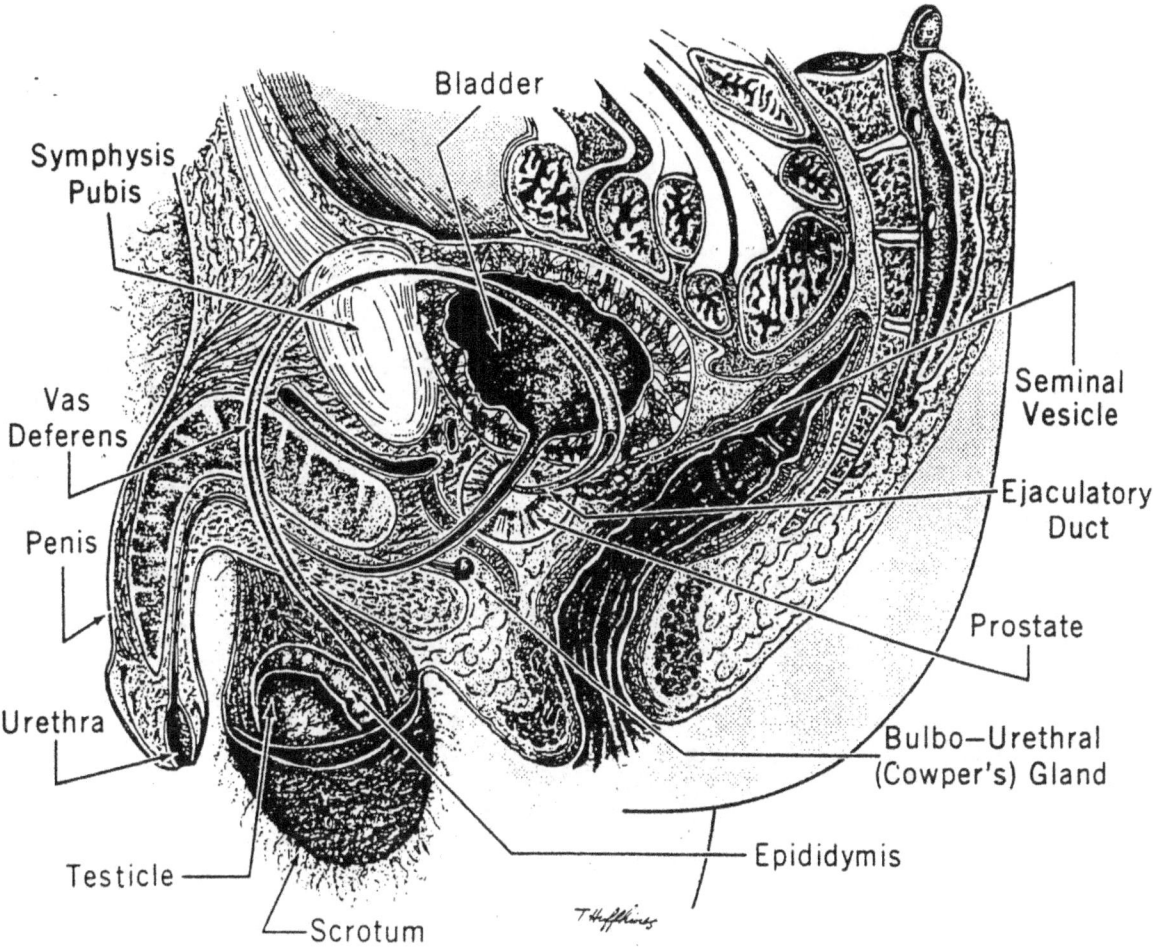

Figure 37. Organs of the Male Reproductive System

duce the female sex cells (ova, or eggs) and the female hormones (estrogen and progesterone). At birth each ovary contains hundreds of potential ova. At puberty, around the age of 12, an ovum matures and is discharged from the ovary. This process is repeated about every 28 days for approximately 30 years. Normally only one ovum matures at a time, with the two ovaries alternating the process at monthly intervals. The discharge of this ovum is called ovulation.

(2) The hormones produced by the ovaries are estrogen and progesterone, which control the sexual development of the female. They are responsible for the form the female body takes, the development of the mammary glands, and the normal functioning of the genital system.

(3) The *fallopian tubes* or, as they are sometimes called, uterine tubes, are two hollow tubes, about 4 inches long, which convey the ovum from an ovary to the uterus.

(4) These tubes lie close to, and partially surround, an ovary, but there is no direct communication between the two. The ovum is actually discharged from an ovary out into the abdominal cavity, where it migrates into the expanded portion of the fallopian tube. The ovum then migrates further into the fallopian tube. If coition has taken place and sperm cells are in the tube, fertilization (union of the male and female sex cells) normally takes place. The "united cell," or the fertilized ovum, then passes through the tube and into the uterus. If no sperm cells are present, the ovum is not fertilized. It fails to develop and disintegrates in its passage to the uterus.

(5) The *uterus* (or womb) is a pear-shaped organ located in the pelvis, between the bladder and the rectum. It is a thick-walled organ measuring about 3 inches in length, 2 inches in width, and 1 inch in thickness in its nonpregnant state. The uterus can be divided into three communicating sections—the fundus, the body, and the cervix. The fundus is the superior portion lying just above the openings for the fallopian tubes. The body is the large, expanded, middle portion. The cervix is the narrow, cylindrical portion just below the uterine body. The cervix is that part of the uterus that protrudes into the vagina. The uterus is held in

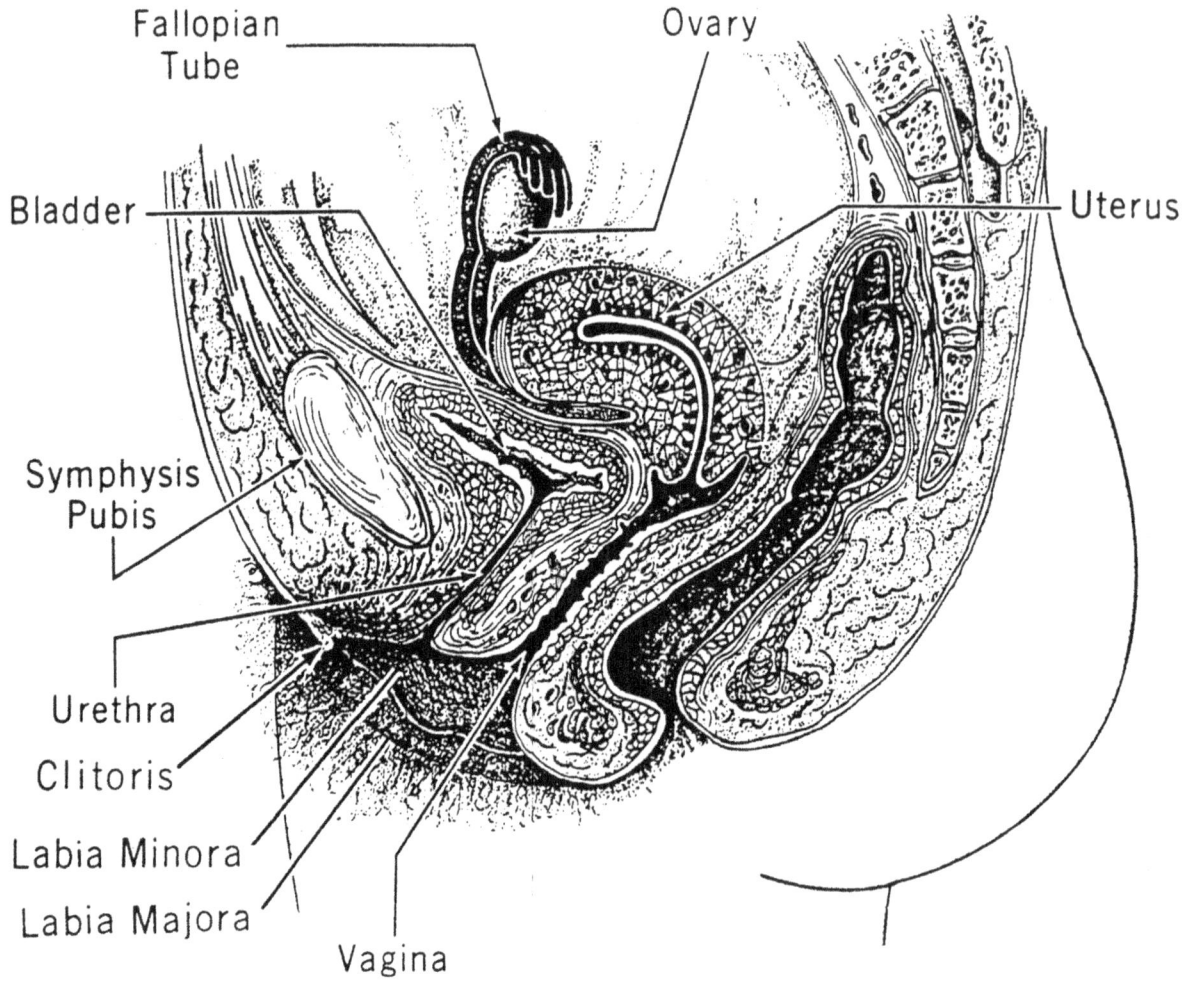

Figure 38. Organs of the Female Reproductive System.

place by several large and strong ligaments. During pregnancy, the uterus increases to several times its normal size, as it houses the unborn child.

(6) The *vagina* is a collapsible musculomembranous canal located between the urethra and the rectum, and behind the urinary bladder. It is about 3 inches in length with its lower opening partially closed by a fold of mucous membrane called the hymen. The hymen covers the vaginal orifice only in the virginal state. The vagina has three essential functions. It serves as an excretory passage for the menstrual flow; it is the female organ of intercourse, receiving the seminal fluid from the male; and it forms the lower part of the birth canal through which the newborn child is delivered. Tissue changes during pregnancy permit the vagina to become greatly distended during the birth of the baby.

(7) The *external genitalia*, collectively referred to as the vulva, include the mons pubis, labia majora, labia minora, clitoris, vestibule, and hymen. Together they serve a secretory and protective function.

(8) The *perineum* is the external surface of the pelvic floor. It includes the area between the anus and the vaginal opening. It is made-up of muscles and fascia which support the pelvic organs. During childbirth this area is often lacerated, or it may be incised to prevent tearing and to facilitate delivery. When a perineal incision is made, the procedure is called an episiotomy.

(9) Anatomically, the breasts, or *mammary glands*, are large, modified skin glands, and belong to the integumentary system. However, their development and function are related to the reproductive system, because their growth and development are regulated by hormones from the ovaries and pituitary glands. The mammary glands undergo noticeable change in the female at puberty, during pregnancy, during and after lactation, and at menopause. Their purpose is milk production for the newborn infant. On occasion, cystic masses occur in breast

tissue, and these, as well as several types of malignant and nonmalignant tumors, are the cause of surgical procedures which range from minor biopsies to radical mastectomies.

(10) *Menstruation* is the periodic sloughing off of the endometrial lining of the uterus. Each month the uterine lining becomes thicker, the blood supply is increased, and hormones are secreted to prepare the uterus for a fertilized ovum. This lining is not needed if the ovum has not been fertilized, and it is expelled through the vagina in the form of a bloody discharge. When an ovum is fertilized and the woman becomes pregnant, the menstrual periods cease until the infant is born.

(11) Pregnancy is that period of time between fertilization and birth, during which the fetus is developing within the uterus. A pregnancy that terminates from premature expulsion of a nonviable fetus is called abortion. Occasionally, the ovum develops outside the uterus, resulting in an ectopic pregnancy. The most common site of an ectopic pregnancy is the fallopian tube. Abortion may necessitate surgical intervention and ectopic pregnancy must be surgically terminated.

c. *Considerations Prior to Surgery*. The surgeon must consider both the hormonal and sex cell functions of the gonads when procedures involving the reproductive organs are being performed.

SECTION K—THE INTEGUMENTARY SYSTEM

48. **The Skin.** Skin is composed of epidermis and dermis. The epidermis is made-up of epithelial tissue. Below this, as can be seen in figure 3-39, is the dermis, which is composed of connective tissue. Located throughout are the various sweat glands and ducts; hair roots and follicles; sebaceous glands; capillaries; and nerve endings for pain, heat, cold, touch, and pressure. The ceruminous glands that secrete earwax, the mammary glands, and the nails are also considered derivatives of the skin.

49. **Functions of the Skin.** The skin excretes waste in sweat, secretes exocrine glandular materials, cools or warms the blood through the dilatation and constriction of capillaries, receives sensory nerve stimulation, and acts as a protective shield against the entrance of infectious agents.

50. **The Healing Process.** Since the majority of surgical procedures require an incision, it is well to

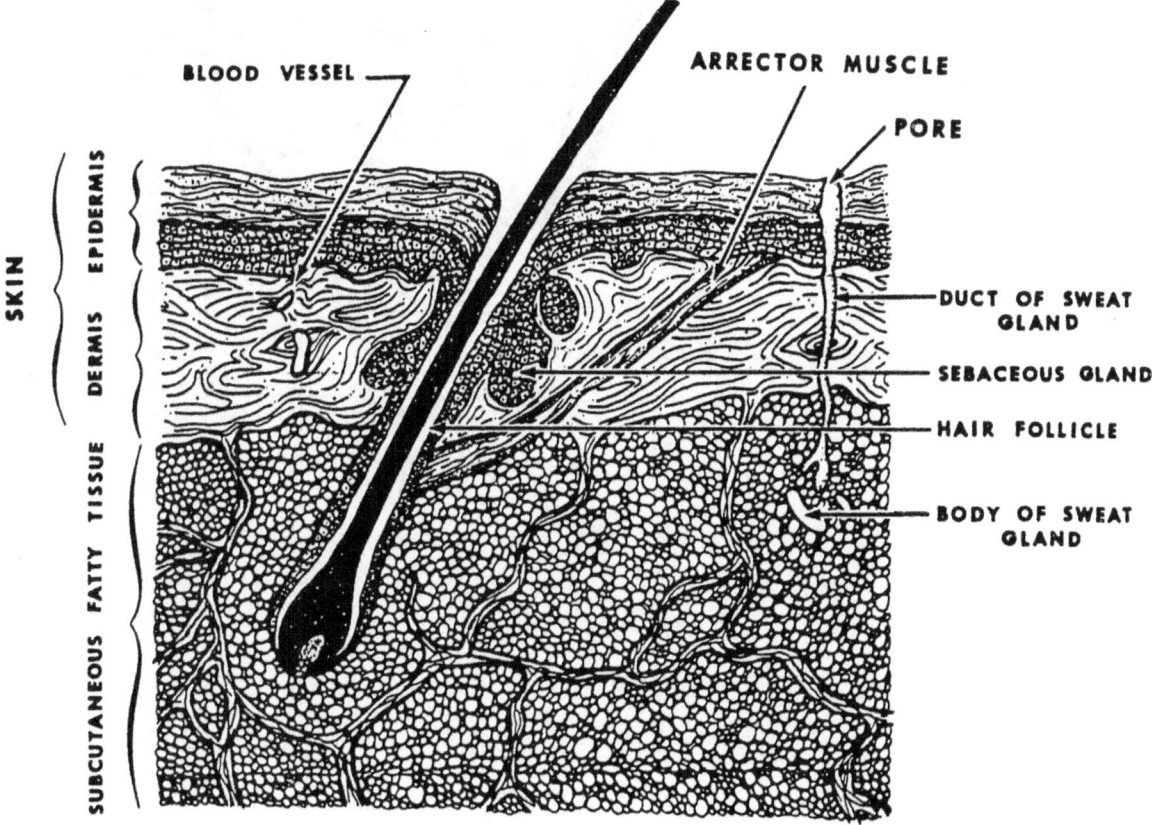

Figure 39. Cross Section of Skin.

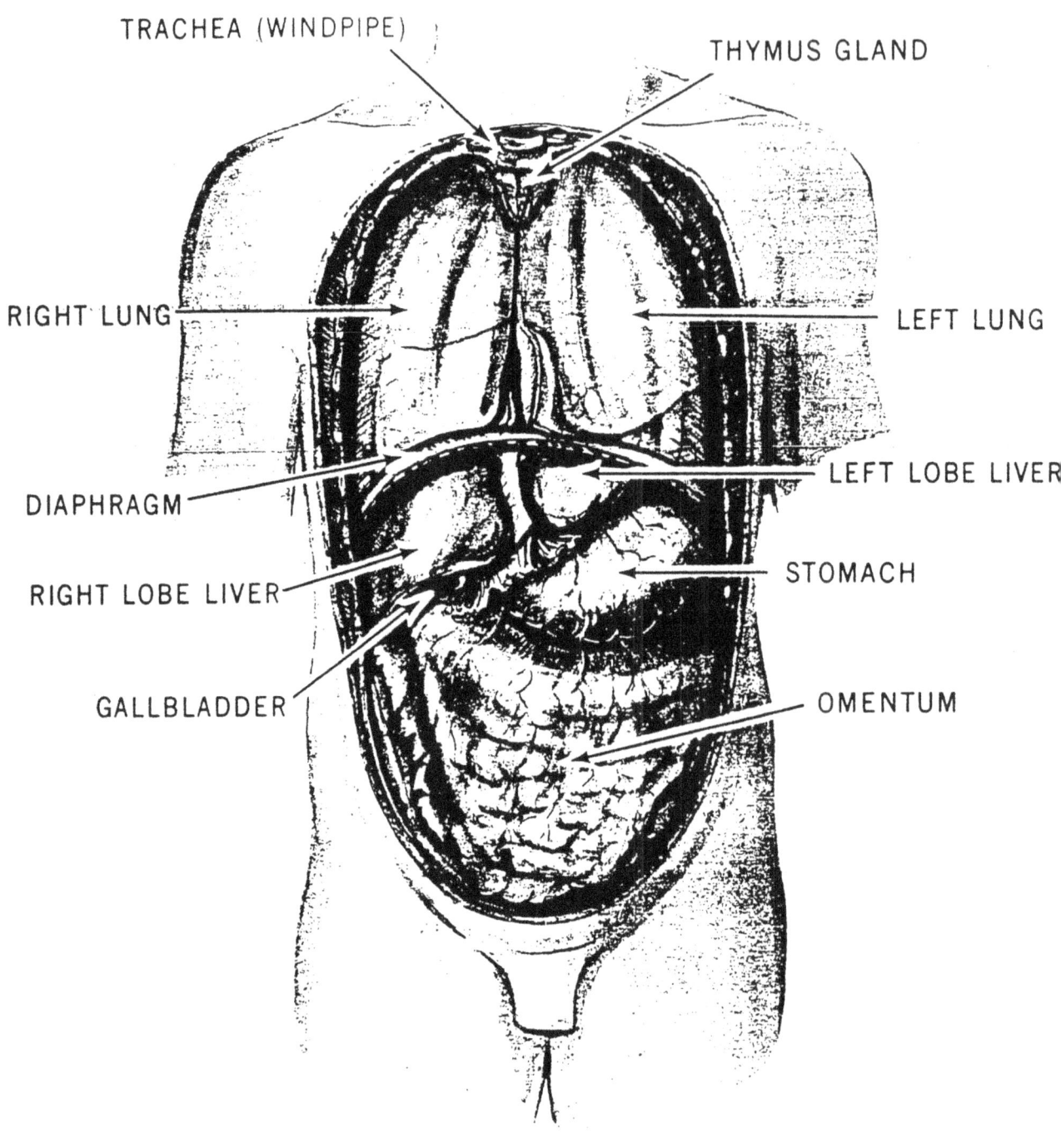

Figure 40. Organs as They Occupy the Thoracic and Abdominal Cavities.

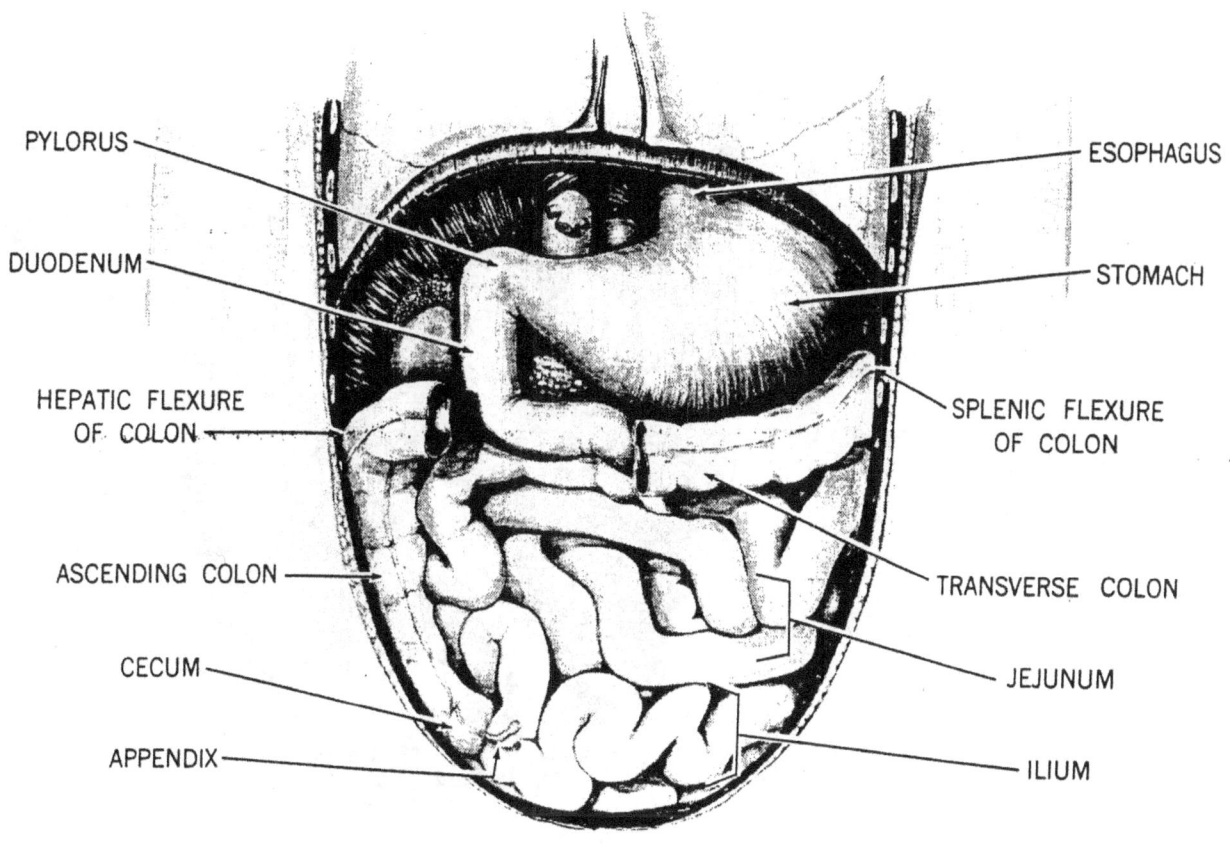

Figure 40. Continued.

know the role of the integumentary system in the healing process and in the formation of scar tissue. The minute bleeding into cut edges and the intact living cells on either side of the incision go through a process whereby new cells are formed. These new cells stretch across the wound and gradually close it. This is called healing by "first intention" or without scar formation. Healing by "second intention" is more common among wounds that have been made by a surgical incision. This involves the filling of the area between the wound edges with granulation tissue formed by the blood and connective tissue cells. This process tends to start in the deeper areas of the wound and work its way toward the surface. This process results in tough, pinkish-gray tissue known as a scar.

SECTION L—THE ORGANS AS THEY OCCUPY THE THORACIC AND ABDOMINAL CAVITIES

51. **Interrelationship and Interdependence of the Body Systems.** The various systems of the body are interrelated and interdependent. Although each is studied separately, it is necessary to understand how they are situated within the body in relationship to each other. See figure 40 which shows the organs as they occupy the thoracic and abdominal cavities and how each structure would be exposed through a thoraco-abdominal incision. The nervous system, the circulatory system, and the numerous layers of connective tissue have been eliminated to provide a clear picture of the internal structures.

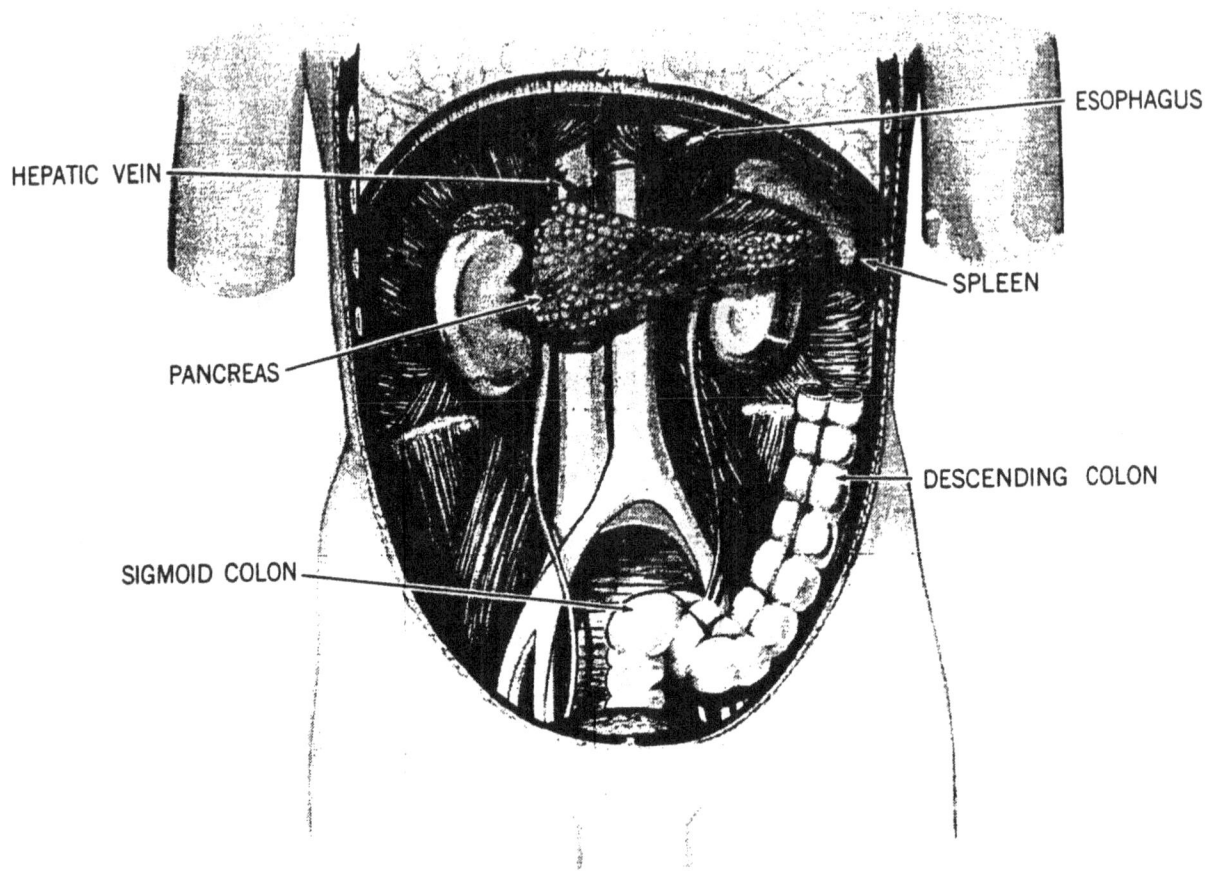

Figure 40. Continued.

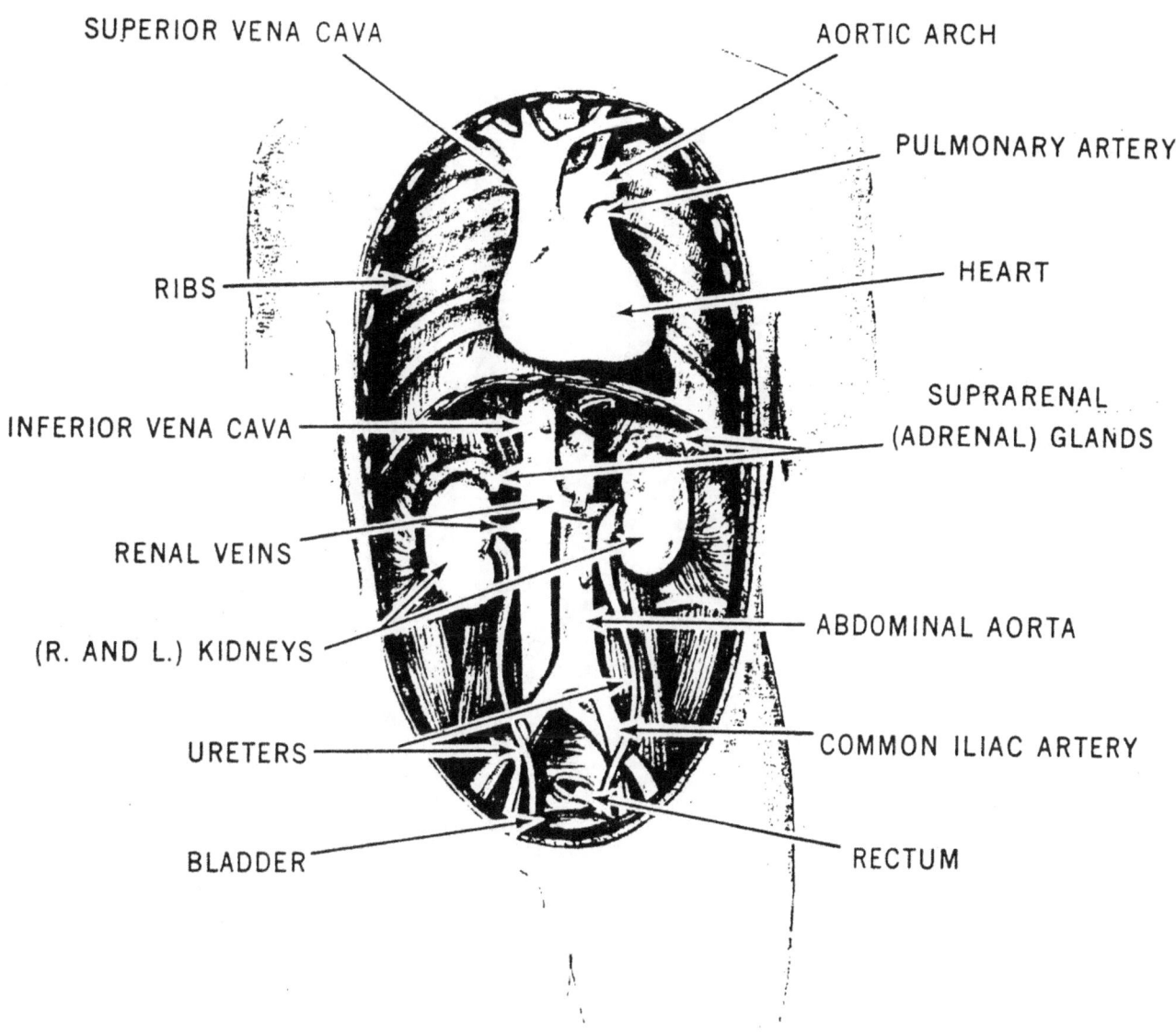

Figure 40. Continued.

FUNERAL SERVICE GLOSSARY

- **ARRANGEMENT ROOM** - A room of the funeral home used to make the necessary funeral arrangements with the family of the deceased.
- **ASPIRATE** - Process of withdrawing fluids and gases from the abdominal cavity.
- **BACKGROUND DRAPES** - Decorative drapes arranged on a frame and placed behind the casket as a background,
- **BEREAVED** - The immediate family of the deceased.
- **BURIAL** - Placing of a dead body in an underground chamber; earth burial; interment.
- **BURIAL CERTIFICATE OR PERMIT** - A legal paper issued by the local government authorizing burial. The permit may authorize earth burial or cremation or removal to a distant point.
- **BURIAL GARMENTS** - Wearing apparel made especially for the dead.
- **BURIAL INSURANCE** - An insurance policy in which the principal is paid in a funeral service and merchandise rather than cash.
- **BURIAL VAULT** - A boxlike container for holding a casket for earth burial; the more substantial vault or a liner is required by most cemeteries to prevent the collapse of a grave after burial.
- **CASH ADVANCE ITEMS** - Goods and services furnished by a third party and paid for by the funeral director on your behalf.
- **CASKET** - A receptacle of wood, metal or plastic into which the dead human body is placed for burial. Sometimes referred to as "coffin" or "burial case."
- **CASKET COACH** - Hearse - A motor coach designed and used for the conveyance of the casketed remains from the place the funeral service is conducted to the cemetery. Also known as a Funeral Coach.
- **CATAFALQUE** - A stand upon which the casketed remains rest while instate and during the funeral service.
- **CEMETERY** - An area of ground set aside for burial or entombment of the deceased.
- **CERTIFIED DEATH CERTIFICATE** - A legalized copy of the original certificate, issued upon request by the local government for the purpose of substantiating various claims by the family of the deceased such as insurance and other death benefits.
- **CHAPEL** - A large room of the funeral home in which the farewell service is held.
- **COFFIN** - A wedge shaped burial case, usually eight-sided.
- **COLUMBARIUM** - A structure of vaults lined with recesses for urns containing cremated remains.
- **COMMITTAL SERVICE** - The final portion of the funeral service at which time the deceased is interred or entombed.
- **COSMETOLOGY** - Utilization of cosmetics to restore life-like appearance to the deceased.
- **CREMAINS** - The remains of a body after cremation; cremated remains.
- **CREMATION** - A process that reduces the body by heat to small bone fragments. When the fragments are pulverized, they are reduced to the consistency of coarse sand or crushed seashells.
- **CREMATORY** - A building with a furnace called a retort which is used to cremate human remains (or the furnace/retort itself)
- **CRYPT** - A vault or room used for keeping remains.
- **DEATH** - Cessation of all vital functions without the capability of resuscitation.

- **DEATH CERTIFICATE** - A legal paper signed by the attending physician showing the cause of death and other vital statistical data pertaining to the deceased.
- **DEATH NOTICE** - A paragraph in the classified section of a newspaper publicizing the death of a person and giving those details of the funeral service the survivors wish to have published. Most such notices list the names of the relatives of the deceased.
- **DECEASED** - (n) one in whom all physical life has ceased; (v) dead.
- **DIRECT BURIAL** - The body is transferred from the place of death to the funeral home, placed in a casket and then delivered directly to the burial site. There is no public viewing or graveside service.
- **DIRECT CREMATION** - The body is transferred from the place of death to the funeral home, placed in a container and delivered directly to a crematory. There is no public viewing.
- **DISPLAY ROOM** - A room in the funeral home in which caskets, urns, burial garments and sometimes vaults are displayed.
- **DISPOSITION** - The final resting place for the body or for cremated remains. Choices include burial of the body in the earth or a mausoleum; burial, scattering or deposit of cremated remains in an urn for placement in a niche or taking home; donation of the body to a research facility; or burial at sea (not permitted in the Great Lakes).
- **EARTH BURIAL** - Interment of a body in a grave.
- **EMBALM** - The process of sanitizing, disinfecting and temporarily preserving a dead body by means of circulating preservative and antiseptic through the veins and arteries.
- **EMBALMER** - One who disinfects or preserves dead human bodies by the injection or external application of antiseptics, disinfectants or preservative fluids; prepares human bodies for transportation which are dead of contagious or infectious diseases; or uses derma surgery or plastic art for restoring mutilated features.
- **EMBALMING FLUID** - Liquid chemicals used in preserving a dead body.
- **EMBALMING TABLE** - An operating table usually constructed of metal with a porcelain surface upon which the remains are placed for embalming.
- **ENTOMBMENT** - Placement of the body in a casket above ground in a mausoleum.
- **FAMILY CAR** - A limousine in the funeral procession set aside for the use of the immediate family.
- **FAMILY ROOM** - A specially arranged room in the funeral home which affords the family privacy at the time of the funeral service.
- **FLOWER CAR** - A vehicle used for the transportation of flower pieces from the funeral home to the church and/or cemetery.
- **FLOWER RACKS AND STANDS** - Wooden or metal stands and racks of varying heights used for banking flowers around the casket.
- **FINAL RITES** - The funeral service.
- **FIRST CALL** - The initial visit of the funeral director to the place of death for the purpose of removing the deceased and to secure certain information for which he has immediate need.
- **FUNERAL ARRANGEMENTS** - Funeral director's conference with the family for the purpose of completing financial and service details of a funeral.
- **FUNERAL DIRECTOR** - A professional who prepares for the burial or other disposition of dead human bodies, supervises such burial or disposition, maintains a funeral establishment for such purposes, counsels with survivors.
- **FUNERAL HOME** - A building used for the purpose of embalming, arranging and conducting funerals.

- **FUNERAL SERVICE** - 1) The profession which deals with the handling of dead human bodies; 2) The religious or other rites conducted immediately before final disposition of the dead human body.
- **FUNERAL SPRAY** - A collective mass of cut flowers sent to the residence of the deceased or to the funeral home as a floral tribute to the deceased.
- **GRAVE** - An excavation in the earth for the purpose of burying the deceased.
- **GRAVE LINER** - A receptacle made of concrete, metal or wood into which the casket is placed as an extra precaution in protecting the remains from the elements. This is required by most cemeteries to prevent the collapse of a grave after burial.
- **GRAVE (OR MEMORIAL) MARKER** - A method of identifying the occupant of a particular grave. Permanent grave markers are usually of metal or stone which gives such data as the name of the individual, date and place of birth, date and place of death.
- **GRAVESIDE SERVICES** - Formal committal services conducted at the cemetery.
- **HONORARY PALLBEARERS** - Friends or members of a religious, social or fraternal organization who act as an escort or honor guard for the deceased. Honorary pallbearers do not carry the casket.
- **IN STATE** - The custom of availing the deceased for viewing by relatives and friends prior to or after the funeral service.
- **INSTRUMENTS** - The varied tools required in the embalming operation.
- **INTER (to)** - To bury a dead body in the earth in a grave or tomb.
- **INTERMENT** - The act of burial.
- **INURNMENT** - The placing of the ashes of one cremated in an urn.
- **LEAD CAR** - The vehicle in which the funeral director and sometimes the clergyman rides. When the procession is formed, the lead car moves to the head of it and leads the procession to the church and/or cemetery.
- **LICENSE** - An authorization from the state granting permission to perform duties that, without such permission, would be illegal.
- **LOWERING DEVICE** - A mechanism used for lowering the casket into the grave. Apparatus is placed over the open grave which has two or more straps which support the casket over the opening. Upon release of the mechanism, the straps unwind from a cylinder and slowly lower the casket into the grave.
- **MAUSOLEUM** - A public or private building especially designed to receive entombments. A permanent above ground resting place for the dead.
- **MARKER** - A monument or memorial to mark the place of burial.
- **MEDICAL EXAMINER** - A government official, usually appointed, who has a thorough medical knowledge and whose function is to perform an autopsy on bodies dead from violence, suicide, crime, etc., and to investigate circumstances of death.
- **MEMORIAL SERVICE** - A religious service conducted in memory of the deceased without the remains being present.
- **MINISTER'S ROOM** - A room in the funeral home set aside for the clergyman wherein he can robe and make any last minute preparations for the funeral service.
- **MORTICIAN** - See funeral director.
- **MORTUARY** - A synonym for funeral home – a building specifically designed and constructed for caring for the dead.
- **MORTUARY SCIENCE** - That part of the funeral service profession dealing with the proper preparation of the body for final disposition.
- **MOURNER** - One who is present at the funeral out of affection or respect for the deceased.

- **NICHE** - A shell-like space in a wall made for the placing of urns containing cremated remains, or inside a building for this purpose (columbarium). Urns are placed in these niches as a final resting place for cremated remains.
- **PALLBEARERS** - Individuals whose duty is to carry the casket when necessary during funeral service.
- **PLOT** - A specific area of ground in a cemetery owned by a family or individual. A plot usually contains two or more graves.
- **PREARRANGED FUNERAL** - Funeral arrangements completed by an individual prior to his/her death.
- **PREARRANGED FUNERAL TRUST** - A method by which an individual can pre-pay their funeral expenses.
- **PREFUNDING** - Same as prearrangement defined above, except that the funding for the funeral is paid in advance either through a trust or life insurance.
- **PRENEED, PREARRANGING or PREPLANNING** - Planning a funeral in advance of the death, usually consisting of a list of your preferences for funeral arrangements.
- **PREPARATION ROOM** - A room in a funeral home designed and equipped for preparing the deceased for final disposition.
- **PREPARATION TABLE** - An operating table located in the preparation room upon which the body is placed for embalming and dressing.
- **PRICE LIST** - An itemized list of funeral goods and services.
- **PROCESSION** - The vehicular movement of the funeral from the place where the funeral service was conducted to the cemetery. May also apply to a church funeral where the mourners follow the casket as it is brought into and taken out of the church.
- **PURGE** - A discharge from the deceased through the mouth, nose and ears of matter from the stomach and intestine caused by improper or ineffectual embalming, due to putrefaction.
- **REGISTER** - A book made available by the funeral director for recording the names of people visiting the funeral home to pay their respects to the deceased. Also has space for entering other data such as name, dates of birth and death of the deceased, name of the officiating clergyman, place of interment, time and date of service, list of floral tributes, etc.
- **REMAINS** - The deceased.
- **REPOSING ROOM** - A room of the funeral home where a body lies in state from the time it is casketed until the time of the funeral service.
- **RESTORATIVE ART** - Derma surgery - The process of restoring mutilated and distorted features by employing wax, creams, plaster, etc.
- **SERVICE CAR** - Usually a utility vehicle to which tasteful ornamentation may be added in the form of a metal firm nameplate, post lamps, etc. It is utilized to transport chairs, church trucks, flower stands, shipping cases, etc.
- **SLUMBER ROOM** - A room equipped with, besides the usual furniture, a bed upon which the deceased is placed prior to casketing on the day of the funeral. The body, appropriately dressed, lies in state on the bed.
- **SPIRITUAL BANQUET** - A Roman Catholic practice involving specific prayers, such as Masses and Rosaries offered by an individual or a group for a definite purpose.
- **SURVIVOR** - The persons outliving the deceased, particularly the immediate family.
- **TRADE EMBALMER** - A licensed embalmer who is not employed by one specific funeral home, but does the embalming for several firms either on a salary or per case basis.

- **TRADITIONAL SERVICE** - A religious service with the body present usually preceded by visitation.
- **TRANSIT PERMIT** - A legal paper issued by the local government authorizing removal of a body to a cemetery for interment. Some cities also require an additional permit if the deceased is to be cremated.
- **URN** - A container into which cremated remains are placed, or in which they are kept; may be made of various materials, including wood, marble or metal.
- **VAULT** - A burial chamber underground or partly so. Also includes in meaning the outside metal or concrete casket container.
- **VIGIL** - A Roman Catholic religious service held on the eve of the funeral service.
- **VISITATION** - A scheduled time, during which a body is present in an open or closed casket, when family and friends pay their respects, usually in private in a special room within the funeral home. Also referred to as a "viewing", "calling hours", "family hour" or "wake."
- **WAKE** - A watch kept over the deceased, sometimes lasting the entire night preceding the funeral.

www.ingramcontent.com/pod-product-compliance
Lightning Source LLC
Chambersburg PA
CBHW081816300426
44116CB00014B/2384